Fundamentals
of
Lung and Heart
Sounds

Fundamentals of Lung and Heart Sounds

THIRD EDITION

Robert L. Wilkins, PhD, RRT, FAARC
Chairman/Professor
Department of Cardiopulmonary Sciences
School of Allied Health Professions
Loma Linda University
Loma Linda, California

John E. Hodgkin, MD
Clinical Professor of Medicine
University of California, Davis
Medical Director, Respiratory Care and Pulmonary Rehabilitation
St. Helena Hospital
Deer Park, California

Brad Lopez, EdD, RRT
Instructor
Health Sciences
Fresno City College
Fresno, California

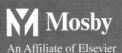

Mosby

An Affiliate of Elsevier

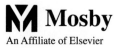

Mosby

An Affiliate of Elsevier

11830 Westline Industrial Drive
St. Louis, Missouri 63146

FUNDAMENTALS OF LUNG AND HEART SOUNDS,
 THIRD EDITION
Copyright © 2004, Mosby, Inc. All rights reserved.

Previous editions copyrighted 1996, 1988.

NOTICE

Pharmacology is an ever-changing field. Standard safety precautions must be
followed, but as new research and clinical experience broaden our knowledge,
changes in treatment and drug therapy may become necessary or appropriate.
Readers are advised to check the most current product information provided by
the manufacturer of each drug to be administered to verify the recommended
dose, the method and duration of administration, and contraindications. It is
the responsibility of the licensed prescriber, relying on experience and knowledge of the patient, to determine dosages and the best treatment for each individual patient. Neither the publisher nor the author assumes any liability for
any injury and/or damage to persons or property arising from this publication.

ISBN-13: 978-0-323-02528-7
ISBN-10: 0-323-02528-5

Managing Editor: Mindy Hutchinson
Senior Developmental Editor: Melissa K. Boyle
Publishing Services Manager: Linda McKinley
Project Manager: Ellen Kunkelmann
Design Manager: Bill Drone
Illustrations in Chapter 3: Stuart Wakefield

Printed in the United States of America

Last digit is the print number: 9 8 7 6 5 4

To our spouses and children

Robert L. Wilkins	*Kristi, Tyler, and Nicholas*
John E. Hodgkin	*Jeanie, Steven, Kathryn, Carolyn, Jonathan, and Jamie*
Brad Lopez	*Jan, Ted, and Justin*

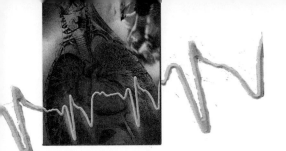

Contributors

James R. Dexter, MD
Chairman, Pulmonary Division
Beaver Medical Group
Redlands, California
Medical Director
Respiratory Care Services
Redlands Community Hospital
Redlands, California
Associate Clinical Professor
Loma Linda University School of Medicine
Loma Linda, California
Chapter 8, Case Studies

Ernie Schwab, PhD
Associate Professor of Allied Health Studies
School of Allied Health Professions
Loma Linda University
Loma Linda, California
Chapter 3, Fundamentals of Sound

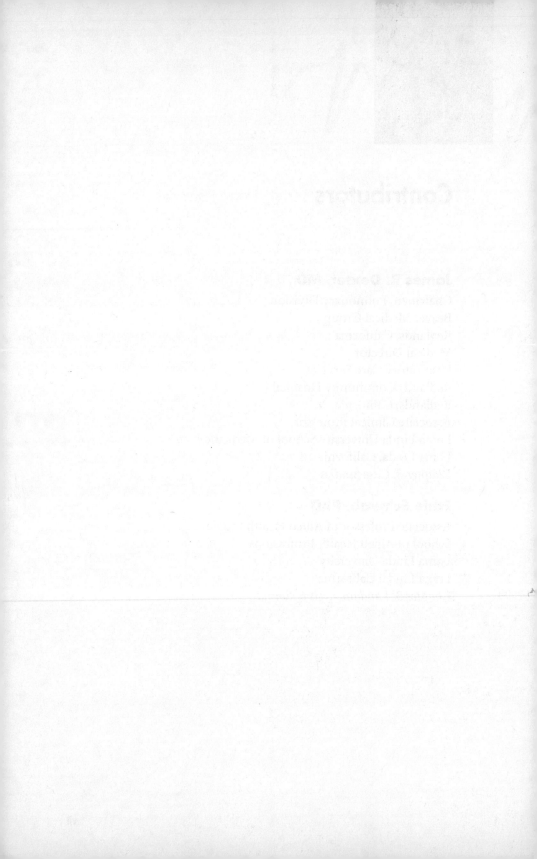

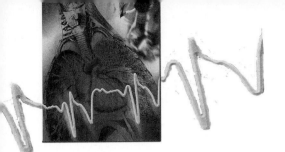

Reviewers

Allen W. Barbaro, MS, RRT

Program Director
Respiratory Care Program
St. Luke's College
Sioux City, Iowa

Regina Clark, MEd, RRT

Program Director
Respiratory Therapy
Northwest Mississippi Community College
Southaven, Mississippi

Nancy A. Davis, RN, BSN

Level III Nurse, Cardiovascular ICU
North Ridge Medical Center
Fort Lauderdale, Florida
Emergency Room
Shands at Live Oak
Live Oak, Florida
Nursing Education Provider
Live Oak, Florida

Sindee Kalminson Karpel, MPA, RRT

Adjunct Professor
Respiratory Therapy Program
Edison Community College
Fort Myers, Florida

Trisha J. Miller, RRT, CPFT, Associate Degree in Applied Science
Respiratory Care Instructor
Carteret Community College
Morehead City, North Carolina

Eric Niegelberg, NREMT-P
Clinical Instructor
Department of Emergency Medicine
EMS Director
Stony Brook University Hospital
Stony Brook, New York

Wilman Ortega, MD
Division of Pulmonary, Critical Care, and Occupational Medicine
SLUCare, St. Louis University Hospital
St. Louis, Missouri

Stanley M. Pearson, MSEd, RRT, C-CPT
Program Director, Respiratory Therapy Technology
College of Applied Sciences and Arts, Health Care Professions
Southern Illinois University—Carbondale
Carbondale, Illinois

Dennis R. Wissing, PhD, CPFT, RRT
Professor of Cardiopulmonary Science
Program Coordinator, Department of Cardiopulmonary Science
Louisiana State University Health Sciences Center
Shreveport, Louisiana

Nancy Wolf
Student, Respiratory Care
Collin County Community College
McKinney, Texas

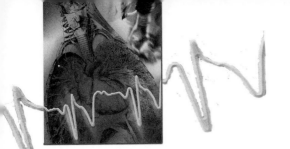

Preface to the Third Edition

Assessment of the patient's heart and lungs represents one of the most important functions performed by health care providers. Abnormalities here must be accurately identified in a timely fashion if patient outcome is to be most favorable. Evaluation of the heart and lungs often centers around auscultation. Chest auscultation provides valuable information about how well the heart and lungs are performing and the specific pathology that may be present. For these reasons, we present this text and audio program with the goal of teaching readers the skill of chest auscultation.

To accomplish the goal of teaching chest auscultation, we begin the book with chapters on pulmonary and cardiac anatomy and physiology. These two chapters were written with the purpose of describing anatomy and physiology as related to the production of heart and lung sounds. Chapter 3 describes the fundamental concepts related to sound physics. Although this topic is not taught traditionally in medically related curriculums, we believe it is vital to a solid understanding of heart and lung sounds. Concepts on the production, conduction, and attenuation of sound are presented. These concepts must be clear to the auscultator if interpretation of the findings is to be accurate and useful. The skills of patient assessment are presented in Chapter 4 with an emphasis on chest examination and auscultation. Chapter 5 describes the history of the stethoscope, presenting information on how the modern stethoscope has evolved over the years. Chapters 6 and 7 are the two most important chapters in the text. Chapter 6 describes vital information on terminology, mechanisms, and interpretation of lung sounds. Chapter 7 does the same for heart sounds. Finally, Chapter 8 presents 10 case studies that illustrate how lung and heart sounds can be most useful in diagnosing the patient. The cases are presented with a description of the history, physical examination, and laboratory data seen upon admission to the outpatient clinic. The lung or heart sounds for each case are presented on the audio program to allow readers to test their diagnostic skills. Each case ends with a series of pertinent questions to test the reader's ability to apply concepts discussed earlier in the text. The answers to the questions are listed at the end of the chapter.

The intended audience of this learning package includes students and practitioners in medicine, nursing, and the allied health professions. Although the text is written at the student level, the experienced clinician will find the content of the text helpful because we present more than the basic information associated with chest auscultation. For example, Chapter 6 describes how to interpret abnormal lung sounds, presents a review of the literature on this topic, and describes how to evaluate the effects of treatment with auscultation.

The first two editions of this text focused strictly on lung sounds. Because many clinicians, such as respiratory therapists, nurses, and paramedics, must be able to assess both the heart and the lungs, we have included both in this edition. Thus the name of the text has been changed to reflect this additional content.

We thank numerous people for their assistance in the production of this text and audio program. The heart sounds were produced by the CardioSim Digital Heart Sound Simulator courtesy of Cardionics, Inc., in Webster, Texas. We thank Keith Johnson at Cardionics for his assistance. We also thank Melissa Boyle and Mindy Hutchinson of Elsevier for their expertise in developing this project into its current form. It has been a joy to work with them.

Readers of this text can receive home study continuing education credits by contacting the author at bob-wilkins@sahp.llu.edu.

Robert L. Wilkins
John E. Hodgkin
Brad Lopez

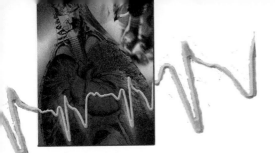

Contents

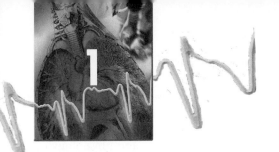

Pulmonary Anatomy and Physiology

OBJECTIVES

After reading this chapter, you will be able to recognize and describe the following:

- Anatomy and physiology of the airways, lung parenchyma, and pleura.
- Pulmonary mechanics and intrathoracic forces that occur during breathing.
- The flow patterns produced in the airways with breathing in health and disease.
- The sound transmission characteristics of healthy lungs.
- The topographic position of lung borders and fissures.

KEY TERMS

diaphragm	respiration	ventilation
parietal pleura	tracheobronchial tree	visceral pleura

INTRODUCTION

The major function of the lungs is gas exchange. On inspiration, atmospheric air enters the airways and travels to the alveoli. Oxygen diffuses from the alveoli through the alveolar-capillary membrane into the blood, and carbon dioxide diffuses from the blood into the alveoli. This is known as external **respiration.** During exhalation, gas moves from the alveoli toward the upper airways and is exhaled through the mouth and nose into the atmosphere. The exchange of air between the lungs and the atmosphere is known as **ventilation.**

This continuous process of ventilation and respiration depends on a patent airway system, intact pulmonary parenchyma, adequate blood flow to the lungs, and a functional neuromuscular system. The purpose of this chapter is to review the anatomy and physiology of the lungs associated with producing lung sounds. Topographic position of the lungs within the chest also is described to assist the reader in learning the appropriate position on the chest wall to best listen for breath sounds.

PULMONARY ANATOMY

Airways

During spontaneous breathing, air enters the upper airways, which consist of the oral and nasal cavities, and pharynx (Figure 1-1). The primary function of the upper airways is to prepare the inspired air for entry into the lungs. The nasal passages act as an "air conditioner." The nasal turbinates and mucous membranes in the nasal cavity warm, filter, and humidify the air during inspiration. Filtering of larger particulates in the inspired air is accomplished in part by the hairs in each nostril. A rich network of blood vessels in the mucosal membrane is instrumental in warming and humidifying the inspired air. While the entire respiratory tract can serve to warm and moisten the inspired air, the nasal passages normally provide the greatest percentage of this function.

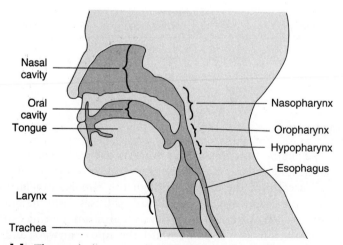

Figure 1-1. The respiratory tract. (*Modified from Hicks GH:* Cardiopulmonary anatomy and physiology, *Philadelphia, 2000, Saunders.*)

The lower airways begin with the larynx. The larynx houses the vocal cords and plays a key role in phonation. Distal to the larynx, the airways can be subdivided into the following three types: 1) the conducting airways, which comprise the trachea and bronchi and end with the terminal bronchioles; 2) the transitional airways, which comprise the respiratory bronchioles, where gas is conducted and some gas exchange occurs; and 3) the alveolar ducts, sacs, and alveoli, where gas exchange takes place with the pulmonary capillary blood.

The trachea, which is about 2.0 to 2.5 cm in diameter and nearly 11 cm long in the adult, extends from the level of the sixth cervical vertebra to the fifth thoracic vertebra. It divides at the level of the carina and forms the right and left mainstem bronchi. The right and left mainstem bronchi further subdivide into lobar bronchi, then segmental bronchi, and then subsegmental bronchi. As the airways become even smaller, they are called *bronchioles*. The larger airways divide into even smaller airways similar to the dichotomous branching of the roots of a tree (Figure 1-2). Collectively, the trachea and branching airways commonly are called the **tracheobronchial tree.**

Each division or generation of airways continues dividing until the airway system reaches the alveoli, the smallest division in the lungs. From the trachea to the alveoli, the airway divides into approximately 23 generations or groups of branching airways in the adult (Figure 1-3).

🖝 Key Point

The entire inhaled volume must pass through the larynx and trachea with each breath. Only a small fraction of this volume passes through each distal bronchus.

Smooth muscle is located in the airway walls throughout most of the tracheobronchial tree, although it varies in its location with the size of the airway. In the trachea and large bronchi, a band of smooth muscle connects the opening of U-shaped cartilages that support the airway. As the airway diameter decreases, the muscle becomes progressively more prominent, with muscle fibers spiraling in both directions. The effect of smooth muscle contraction (bronchoconstriction or bronchospasm) is more significant distal to the trachea and large bronchi and will decrease airway diameter and length. Smooth muscle is present in airway walls to the level of the respiratory bronchioles.

The smooth muscles that line the airway walls may contract in response to various stimuli. Dust, cold air, pollen, and infection are

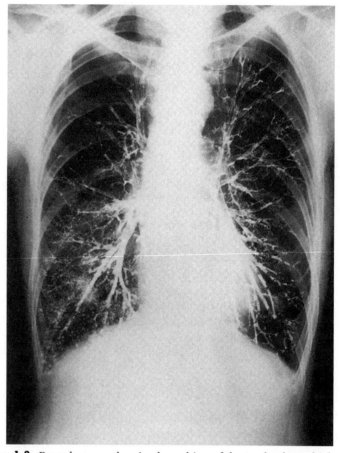

Figure 1-2. Bronchogram showing branching of the tracheobronchial tree.

common causes of bronchospasm. Patients with asthma have hyper-activity of the airways and are prone to periods of labored breathing and extreme shortness of breath. Airflow in the airways of these patients is initially more rapid and turbulent in comparison with the patient with healthy airways. If the patient fatigues, the flow pattern within the airways will slow and become less turbulent.

Ciliated columnar epithelial cells line nearly the entire respiratory tract from the larynx to the level of the respiratory bronchioles. The cilia that border the columnar epithelium constantly wave back and forth in a rhythmic pattern similar to what is seen as the wind blows over a wheat field. This process removes most of the particles and debris entrapped in the mucus. The mucociliary "escalator" does an effective job of keeping the airways clean.

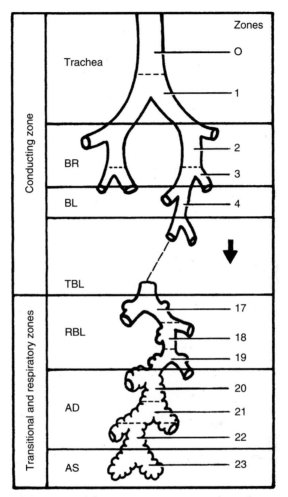

Figure 1-3. Subdivisions of the respiratory tract: *BR*, bronchus; *BL*, bronchiole; *TBL*, terminal bronchiole; *RBL*, respiratory bronchiole; *AD*, alveolar duct; *AS*, alveolar space.

Lung Parenchyma and Sound Transmission

The lung parenchyma is made up of millions of alveoli surrounded by a rich network of pulmonary capillaries. The close interface between the alveolar walls and pulmonary capillaries allows for gas exchange between the lungs and the blood. The parenchyma also contains many air-filled airways that carry the inhaled air to the distal lung units. As a result, the healthy lungs are very low-density organs that float when placed in water. Hyperinflation of the lungs will decrease the density further, whereas diseases that consolidate the lungs (e.g., pneumonia and pulmonary edema) increase the density.

Sound waves, especially high-frequency waves, are known to travel poorly through low-density matter and better through high-density matter (see Chapter 3). This point can be illustrated easily by connecting two tin cans by a long string of wire. The sounds spoken into one can rapidly pass through the dense wire to the other can. Although the exact words spoken into the first can are not appreciated in the second can, the sound vibrations are readily present. Now replace the wire with a low-density material (such as string), and the sound vibrations will not pass from one can to the next nearly as well because of attenuation. The healthy lung is a low-density structure.

☞ Key Point

High-frequency sound vibrations are attenuated (diluted) by the low-density structures (e.g., lungs) and less attenuated by high-density structures.

The Pleura

The lungs are surrounded closely by two membranes: the **visceral pleura,** which attaches to the lungs, and the **parietal pleura,** which attaches to the chest wall. A thin layer of fluid, present between the two layers of the pleura, lubricates the membranes and provides frictionless movement of the lungs against the chest wall with breathing. The fluid in the pleural space also provides molecular cohesive forces that prevent separation of the lungs from the chest wall under normal circumstances. This allows the lungs to follow the direction of the chest wall and diaphragm with breathing.

The pleural space is normally very thin and not a significant issue in the transmission of sound from within the chest through the chest wall. Abnormalities that cause a build-up of fluid, blood, or air in the pleural space influence the passage of sound through the chest wall (see Chapters 4 and 6).

MECHANICS OF BREATHING

The Chest Wall

The human thorax is rigid and structured to protect the vital organs contained within yet flexible and pliable enough to permit chest expansion with breathing. The bones, cartilage, and supportive tissue provide sufficient rigidity and strength to the thorax, whereas the numerous points of articulation allow significant changes in size and shape. The 12 pairs of ribs provide the structural foundation of the chest (Figure 1-4).

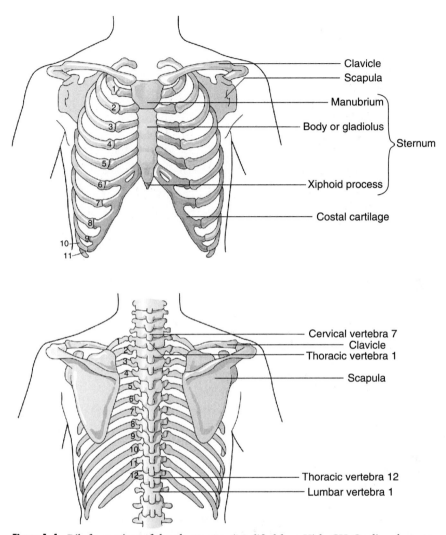

Figure 1-4. Rib formation of the chest cage. *(Modified from Hicks GH:* Cardiopulmonary anatomy and physiology, *Philadelphia, 2000, Saunders.)*

During inspiration, the chest and lungs expand in all three planes: anteroposterior, transverse, and longitudinal. The three-dimensional increase in the size of the chest occurs because the ribs move anteriorly and upward, spreading apart as a result of the contraction of the diaphragm and accessory muscles of inspiration.

Muscles of Respiration

The muscles used in breathing can be divided into two components: primary and accessory (Figure 1-5). The primary muscle of respiration

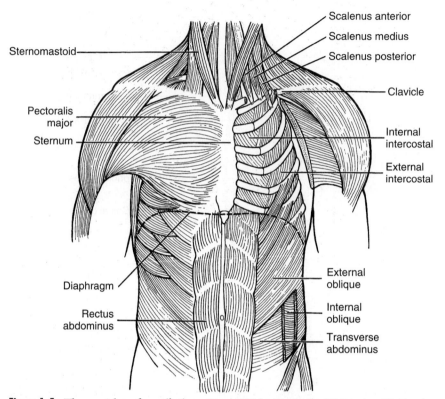

Figure 1-5. The muscles of ventilation. *(From Wilkins RL, Stoller JK, Scanlan CL:* Egan's fundamentals of respiratory care, *ed 8, St Louis, 2003, Mosby.)*

is the **diaphragm,** which consists of two dome-shaped hemidiaphragms that form the floor of the thorax and separate it from the abdomen. During inspiration, the diaphragm contracts and descends toward the abdomen. Diaphragmatic contraction causes the longitudinal lung size to increase. During exhalation, the diaphragm relaxes and ascends because of lung recoil and returns to its resting, dome-shaped configuration.

Accessory muscles of breathing, located in the neck and upper part of the chest, can assist the diaphragm in increasing thoracic volume. Accessory muscles of breathing include sternocleidomastoid, the scalenes, intercostals, pectoralis major, external oblique, and abdominal muscles (see Figure 1-5). These muscles normally are not active during relaxed breathing but begin participating in breathing with heavy activity or when the work of breathing is increased. Rapid breathing with exercise, cardiopulmonary diseases, or any problem that increases the work of breathing often causes the accessory muscles of breathing to become active to augment ventilation. The accessory muscles can increase the magnitude of chest expansion and lung size that occurs during inspiration.

☞ Key Point

Significant lung disease causes the accessory muscles of breathing to become active. These muscles increase ventilation by lifting the anterior portion of the rib cage, thus increasing A-P diameter with each breath.

The abdominal muscles usually do not participate actively in relaxed breathing; however, during forced exhalation, rapid breathing, exercise, coughing, or sneezing, the abdominal muscles play an important part in providing maximal function. They are especially important in post-operative patients who must use them to generate an effective cough or in patients with lung diseases that cause excessive airway secretions.

How Breathing Occurs

From a mechanical point of view, the lungs and surrounding chest wall form the ventilatory apparatus that is similar in function to a pump. During inspiration, the diaphragm contracts and the lungs expand as a result of the pressure in the pleural space and distal lung units becoming increasingly subatmospheric. The pressure gradient created between the airway opening at the mouth and alveoli causes air from the atmosphere to fill the lungs. Toward the end of inspiration, the volume of air in the lungs increases; alveolar pressure approximates atmospheric pressure; and air flow into the lungs stops. During exhalation, as the inspiratory muscles relax and the lungs recoil, alveolar pressure now exceeds pressure at the airway opening. This pressure gradient causes air to flow out of the lungs. Exhalation ends when the pressure gradient between the alveoli and upper airway equilibrates. The pumping action created by alternating changes in lung pressure provides lung ventilation essential to life (Figure 1-6).

The swings in pleural and distal lung pressure that occur with breathing influence airway patency contained within the lungs. As the pleural pressure decreases with inspiration, the airways are "pulled" open and expand to a more patent position. The opposite is true during exhalation. During exhalation, the airway walls recoil inward to a more narrow resting position. This change in airway caliber with breathing is not clinically significant under normal conditions. When the airways are narrowed, as with asthma and chronic obstructive pulmonary disease (COPD), the variance in airway caliber is often significant and explains why patients with obstructive lung disease

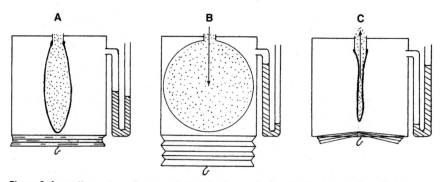

Figure 1-6. Balloon-in-a-box model of the lung-thorax. **A,** In the resting position, a small negative pressure in the box keeps the balloon slightly distended. **B,** As the box expands, the cavity becomes more negative, and air flows into the balloon. **C,** If the floor of the box is pushed upward, positive pressure develops in the box, and the balloon empties more completely. *(From Spearman CB, Sheldon RL, Egan DF: Egan's fundamentals of respiratory care, ed 4, St Louis, 1982, Mosby.)*

have trouble exhaling. Narrowing of the intrathoracic airways during exhalation worsens the obstruction and makes it clinically important. This concept is exaggerated during forceful breathing. Maximal inspiratory effort opens intrathoracic airways maximally while forceful exhalation causes dynamic compression of the airways. Such forceful breathing occurs during heavy exercise in healthy people but at rest in those with asthma during episodes of severe airways obstruction.

☞ Key Point

Intrathoracic airways tend to expand open during inhalation and narrow during exhalation. The changes in airway caliber with breathing are exaggerated during forceful (labored) breathing.

Breathing Control

The rate and depth of breathing are initiated and controlled by the brain. Both the voluntary and involuntary nervous system influence the breathing pattern. The cerebral cortex controls voluntary breathing rate and volume, and the ventral and lateral parts of the medulla oblongata control involuntary breathing. Voluntary and involuntary inspiration occurs when the phrenic nerve stimulates contraction of the diaphragm, thus causing air to enter the airways and the lung to expand. Expiration is passive. Damage to certain parts of the brain will influence the patient's breathing pattern and thus the quality of breath sounds heard. Breathing may become deep and fast or slow and shallow with brain injury or disease. The resulting breath sounds will vary accordingly; they become louder with deep breathing and softer with shallow breathing.

The diameter of the airways is partially controlled by stimulation of the involuntary nerves that innervate the smooth muscles in the airways. Stimulation of the sympathetic nervous system leads to relaxation of the smooth muscle and an increase in airway diameter. Conversely, stimulation of the cholinergic system leads to airway narrowing. Airflow and turbulence in the airways are altered by changes in the airway diameter (Figure 1-7).

Laminar

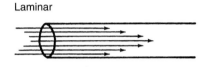

Turbulent

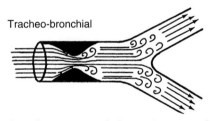

Tracheo-bronchial

Figure 1-7. Types of air flow. In smooth, large airways, turbulent flow occurs at high velocities; this is common in the trachea and main bronchi, especially with hyperpnea (hyperventilation). The flow rate in the small airways is very low because the total air flow is divided among many airways. However, eddy formation may occur at each branching of the tracheo-bronchial tree, and the pressure required for eddy flow is approximately the same as for turbulent flow. Turbulence (at low flow rates) or eddy formation is particularly apt to occur where there are irregularities—such as those caused by mucus, exudate, tumor or foreign bodies, or partial closure of the glottis—in the tubes. Sometimes air flow is a combination of laminar and turbulent flow with eddy formation. *(Redrawn from Forster RE II et al: The lung: physiologic basis of pulmonary function tests, ed 3, St Louis, 1986, Mosby.)*

CHEST TOPOGRAPHY

Anterior-Posterior View

An anterior view of the lungs shows the apex of each lung extending from the base of the neck above the clavicle near the vertebral end of the first rib, down to the sixth rib at the midclavicular line (Figure 1-8).

The right lung is divided into the upper and middle lobe by the horizontal fissure, which begins near the fourth rib anteriorly at the midsternal line and continues laterally to the fifth rib at the midaxillary line. The oblique fissure of the right lung separates the lower lobe from the upper and middle lobes. It extends from the sixth rib anteriorly at the midclavicular line and ascends to the fourth rib posteriorly (Figures 1-8 and 1-9). The oblique fissure for the left lung separates the lower lobe from the upper lobe. It occupies a position similar to the oblique fissure of the right lung. The breath sounds of the upper lobes of both lungs and the right middle lobe dominate the auscultation findings heard over the anterior chest.

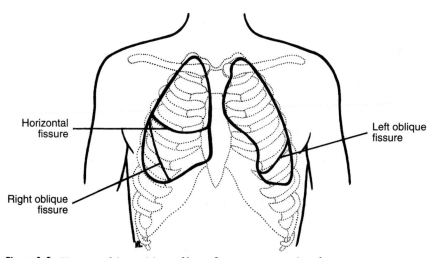

Horizontal fissure

Left oblique fissure

Right oblique fissure

Figure 1-8. Topographic position of lung fissures on anterior chest. *(From Wilkins RL, Krider SJ, Sheldon RL: Clinical assessment in respiratory care, ed 4, St Louis, 2000, Mosby.)*

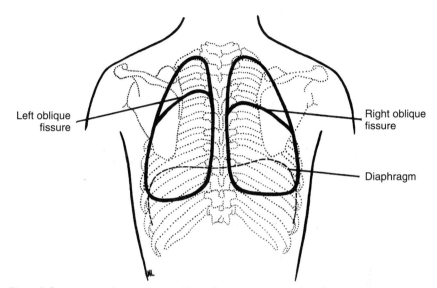

Figure 1-9. Topographic position of lung fissures on posterior chest. *(From Wilkins RL, Krider SJ, Sheldon RL: Clinical assessment in respiratory care, ed 4, St Louis, 2000, Mosby.)*

☞ Key Point

The right middle lobe is best assessed on the anterior chest wall.

Posterior-Anterior View

From a posterior-to-anterior view, the lungs are divided into upper and lower lobes by the oblique fissures. The oblique fissure originates near T-3 at the midspinal line and extends anteriorly to the level of the sixth rib. The lower lobes dominate the surface area of the posterior chest wall. The upper lobes can be auscultated posteriorly above the midlevel of the scapula or above T-3 (see Figure 1-9).

☞ Key Point

The lower lobes of the left and right lungs are best assessed on the posterior chest.

Lateral View

The lateral aspect of the chest is an excellent place to evaluate the lungs because of the limited muscle and bony interference. The inferior margin of the lung is located at the eighth rib at the midaxillary line in healthy individuals at rest. The inferior margin moves downward with deep inspiratory effort and upward with full expiratory effort. Evaluation of the lateral aspect of the chest can extend upward to the apex of the axilla.

ALTERATIONS IN THE LUNGS WITH CHEST DISEASE

Many chest diseases can be classified as *restrictive* or *obstructive* lung disorders or a combination of the two. Restrictive lung diseases cause a reduction in lung volume and result in less air within the lung; thus the lung density increases with restrictive diseases. Obstructive lung disorders primarily affect the airways and alveoli, thus resulting in diminished airflow. Air trapping often occurs with obstructive lung disease, thus resulting in hyperinflation of the distal air spaces and a decrease in lung density. Obstructive lung disease often causes an increase in the production of mucus in the lower airways. This mucus may narrow further the airways and change the dynamics of flow within. Mucus also may produce unique sounds as air passes by and interfaces with it (see Chapter 6).

Restrictive and obstructive lung diseases cause dramatic changes in pulmonary anatomy and physiology. Many of these changes can be detected on physical examination, including significant alterations in lung sounds, as discussed in Chapter 6.

☞ Key Point

Restrictive lung disease causes the lung to increase in density and obstructive lung disease with hyperinflation causes the lung to decrease in density. These changes in the lung alter the sound transmission characteristics of the lung (see Chapter 3).

Chapter Highlights

- The upper airway consists of the mouth, nose, oral pharynx, and nasal pharynx. Their primary purpose is to prepare the inhaled gas for entry into the lung.
- The lower airway begins with the larynx and trachea. It contains 23 divisions of airways that terminate in the respiratory bronchioles, alveolar ducts, and alveolar sacs.
- The normal lungs are low-density structures that conduct sound waves poorly (see Chapter 3).
- The lungs are connected to the chest wall by pleural membranes. The parietal pleura are attached to the chest wall and the visceral pleura to the lung. A small layer of fluid is present between the two membranes and reduces friction between the lung and chest wall with breathing. This fluid also provides molecular cohesive force that prevents separation of the lung from the chest wall.

- The tight connection between the layers of the pleura allows the lungs to follow the direction of the chest wall and diaphragm with breathing. Excess fluid or air in the space between the two layers of the pleura alters the ability of sounds from within the chest to be heard on the surface of the chest.
- The diaphragm is the primary muscle of breathing. Contraction of the diaphragm causes a drop in the distal lung pressure. This causes air to flow into the airways. Exhalation occurs when the diaphragm relaxes and the lungs recoil back to their resting position. This causes an increase in alveolar pressure relative to mouth pressure, and gas moves outward.
- The horizontal fissure separates the right middle lobe from the right upper lobe. It runs from the fourth rib on the anterior chest at the sternal border to the fifth rib at the midaxillary line.
- The oblique fissure separates the upper lobe from the lower lobe on the posterior chest wall. It runs laterally from T-3 at the midspinal line on the posterior chest.
- Restrictive lung disease increases the density of the affected lung, and obstructive lung disease with hyperinflation decreases lung density. Sound transmission through the lung is altered by such pathology.

BIBLIOGRAPHY

- Beachey W: *Respiratory care anatomy and physiology: foundations for clinical practice,* St Louis, 1998, Mosby.
- Hicks G: *Cardiopulmonary anatomy and physiology,* Philadelphia, 2000, WB Saunders.

Review Questions

1. What term is used to describe gas exchange between the lung and the pulmonary circulation?
   A. Ventilation
   B. Internal respiration
   C. External respiration
   D. Oxygenation

2. What structure is considered the first part of the lower airway?
   A. Pharynx
   B. Larynx
   C. Trachea
   D. Bronchi

3. What cells line the lower airways and are responsible for physically removing dust and debris inhaled into the lung?
   A. Goblet cells
   B. Mucous cells

Continued

Review Questions—cont'd

    C. Smooth muscle cells
    D. Ciliated columnar epithelial cells

4. True or False
    The normal lung transmits high-frequency sounds poorly.

5. True or False
    Smooth muscle contraction in the airways does little to alter tracheal patency.

6. True or False
    The accessory muscles of breathing are active even at rest in the healthy person.

7. What factor normally causes the diaphragm to ascend back to its resting position after contraction?
    A. Lung recoil
    B. Abdominal muscle contraction
    C. Negative intrathoracic pressure
    D. None of the above

8. True or False
    Distal airways tend to open during inhalation and narrow during exhalation.

9. True or False
    Stimulation of the sympathetic nervous system leads to bronchoconstriction.

10. The horizontal fissure begins at what rib at the midsternal line?
    A. Rib 2
    B. Rib 4
    C. Rib 6
    D. Rib 8

11. True or False
    The lower lobes are best assessed laterally.

12. True or False
    Restrictive lung diseases tend to cause a loss of lung volume and an increase in lung density.

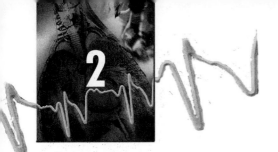

Cardiac Anatomy and Physiology

OBJECTIVES

After reading this chapter, you will be able to recognize and describe the following:
- The four chambers of the heart and the function of each.
- What is meant by the left side of the heart being a high-pressure system.
- The four cardiac valves and the function of each.
- The definition of cardiac output and the three major factors that determine it.
- The topographic position of the heart in the chest.

KEY TERMS

afterload	diastole	stroke volume
cardiac output	ejection fraction	systole
contractility	preload	

INTRODUCTION

The purpose of this chapter is to describe the anatomy and physiology of the heart as it pertains to cardiac auscultation. The structures associated with producing or affecting heart sounds will be emphasized. In addition, because an understanding of the position of the heart within the chest is vitally important to the process of cardiac auscultation, cardiac topography will be presented.

THE HEART

The heart is a four-chambered organ that pumps blood throughout the body. It is useful to view the heart as having two sides: the left and the right. The left side is made up of the left atrium and left ventricle. The left atrium receives oxygenated blood from the pulmonary veins and pumps this blood into the left ventricle. The left ventricle has the important job of pumping oxygenated blood (arterial blood) to all areas of the body for the purpose of maintaining tissue oxygenation to sustain life. Once the arterial blood gives up some of its oxygen and takes on carbon dioxide, it becomes venous blood and returns to the right side of the heart via the veins.

The left side of the heart is a high-pressure system. Pressures generated in the left ventricle reach a high of approximately 120 mm Hg during contraction in the healthy heart. The left ventricle must generate such pressure because it pushes arterial blood to all parts of the body. For this reason, the arterial circulation is also a high-pressure system in comparison with the venous circulation.

The right side of the heart also comprises two chambers: the right atrium and the right ventricle. The right side of the heart is a low-pressure system under normal conditions. The right atrium receives venous blood from the superior and inferior vena cava and pumps it into the right ventricle. The right ventricle serves to pump the deoxygenated blood to the pulmonary circulation and lungs where fresh oxygen is available. The peak pressure in the right ventricle during contraction is only about 25 mm Hg normally. Once the blood has been oxygenated, it returns to the left atrium and left ventricle for recirculation to the arterial system.

The heart performs its duties through a continuous and coordinated process of contracting and relaxing. First both atria contract, which after a short pause (0.2 seconds) is followed by the simultaneous contraction of both ventricles. Ventricular contraction is also called **systole** and ventricular relaxation is known as **diastole.** Each systole results in a certain volume of blood ejected into the aorta (left side) or pulmonary artery (right side). The amount of blood ejected with each systole by the left ventricle is known as the stroke volume (the volume ejected by the right ventricle should be the same as the volume ejected by the left ventricle in healthy people). The diastolic period allows the ventricles to fill with blood before contraction. Early in diastole the ventricles fill passively with the blood that has collected in the atria during the previous ventricular contraction. Late in diastole the ventricles fill due to atrial contraction. This is known as the *atrial kick,* and it boosts the ventricular end-diastolic volume to an optimal level just prior to systole.

☞ Key Point

Ventricular filling occurs during diastole in two ways: initially because of passive blood flow from the atria and subsequently from atrial contraction just before systole.

Heart Valves

Both sides of the heart contain two one-way valves for a total of four. The right atrium is separated from the right ventricle by the tricuspid valve (Figure 2-1). This valve opens during diastole and allows blood to flow from the right atrium to the right ventricle. It closes during systole as pressure builds in the right ventricle and serves to stop blood from flowing backwards into the right atrium.

Flow from the right ventricle into the pulmonary artery occurs through the pulmonic valve (see Figure 2-1). This valve opens during systole to allow blood to flow from the right ventricle into the pulmonary artery. It closes during diastole as pressure in the right ventricle drops and prevents the backflow of blood from the pulmonary artery into the right ventricle.

On the left side of the heart, the left atrium is separated from the left ventricle by the mitral valve (also known as the bicuspid valve) (see Figure 2-1). This valve opens during diastole and allows blood to flow smoothly into the left ventricle under normal circumstances. It closes during systole to prevent the backflow of blood into the left atrium. The mitral valve must be structurally sound because of the high pressure to which it is exposed during each systolic contraction of the powerful left

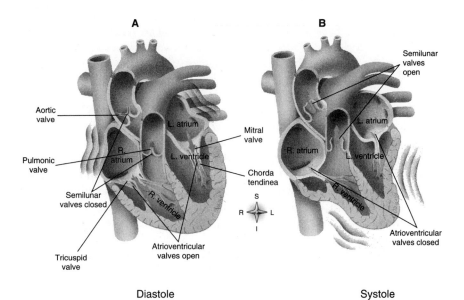

Figure 2-1. Anatomy of the heart, showing the four heart valves and their position during diastole (**A**) and systole (**B**). *(Modified from Thibodeau GA, Patton KT: Anatomy and physiology, ed 5, St Louis, 2003, Mosby.)*

ventricle. Defects in this valve are of major concern because they could lead to inadequate circulation of oxygenated blood to the body. If the left ventricular output and blood pressure drop significantly, a condition known as *shock* occurs, and tissue hypoxia is likely.

Blood flow out of the left ventricle passes through the aortic valve and then into the aorta (see Figure 2-1). The aortic valve opens during systole and closes during diastole. Its closure during diastole prevents the backflow of oxygenated blood into the left ventricle. This valve also is under high pressure during diastole and must be structurally sound to prevent arterial blood from regurgitating back into the left ventricle.

The one-way heart valves open and close because of pressure changes. Increased pressure on the proximal side of the valve causes it to open; increasing pressure on the distal side causes it to close. The valves are not influenced directly by the nervous system. The pressure changes from one side of a valve to the other, however, may be influenced indirectly by sympathetic and parasympathetic stimulation. For example, sympathetic activity causes the heart to beat faster and the myocardium to contract more forcefully, which may then cause changes in the pressure within the heart.

☞ Key Point

Heart valves open and close in response to pressure changes from one side to the other. They primarily serve to prevent the backflow of blood in the wrong direction. The pressure forcing the valve shut varies with many factors, such as blood pressure and strength of ventricular contraction.

The heart valves located between the atria and the ventricles are collectively known as the *A-V valves* (atrioventricular valves). The A-V valves typically move in simultaneous or near simultaneous fashion, opening during diastole and closing during systole (see Figure 2-1). The valves located at the opening of the aorta and pulmonary artery are collectively known as the *semilunar valves*. The semilunar valves also work in a coordinated fashion opening and closing at nearly the same instant. They open during systole and close during diastole (see Figure 2-1).

An important feature of the A-V valves is the chordae tendinae. Chordae tendinae are fibrous strands that are connected to papillary muscles on one end and to the edges and ventricular surfaces of the mitral or tricuspid valves on the other end. These small tendinous cords prevent the inversion of the A-V valves during systole. Closure and competence of the A-V valves can be affected by damage to the valve leaflets or to the papillary muscles and chordae tendinae.

The Pericardium

The pericardium is a saclike structure that surrounds the heart. It comprises an inner layer (visceral) that attaches to the heart and an outer layer (parietal) that attaches to a fibrous membrane, known as the *fibrous pericardium* (Figure 2-2). The potential space between the visceral and parietal layers of the pericardium is known as the pericardial cavity. Normally this space contains a small amount of fluid that provides lubrication to permit smooth, low-friction movement of the heart. This function of the pericardium is similar to the action of the visceral and parietal layers of the pleura, which also contain a small amount of fluid for ease of lung movement.

Normally, the pericardium does not produce any sounds with movement of the heart and does not significantly attenuate any sounds coming from within the heart. If the pericardium fills with fluid, however, the heart sounds may not be heard on the surface of the chest wall or they may be muffled. In addition, inflammation of the pericardium may result in friction sounds that occur with movement of the heart, especially during systole (see Chapter 7).

CARDIAC OUTPUT

The amount of blood pumped out of the left ventricle per minute is known as the **cardiac output.** Cardiac output is a function of the heart rate multiplied by the **stroke volume.** Stroke volume is determined by three important factors: preload, afterload, and contractility. Abnormalities in any one of these factors can lead to a poor cardiac output and shock. **Preload** is defined as the amount of ventricular filling during diastole. Inadequate filling of the heart before contraction (low preload) is common with hypovolemia. Overstretching of the heart is seen with hypervolemia and is common in heart failure patients because they retain water in response to decreased renal perfusion. In either case the heart cannot pump blood effectively if the preload is too high or too low.

Afterload is a measure of the resistance to flow out of the ventricle. This resistance also must be at an optimal level. Too little resistance causes a drop in blood pressure and inadequate perfusion of vital organs. Afterload that is too high causes blood flow out of the ventricles to be less than optimal. Afterload for the right side of the heart is determined by pulmonary vascular resistance (PVR). PVR increases when pulmonary vasoconstriction occurs such as when hypoxia is present in part of or all of the lung. Afterload for the left side of the heart is a function of systemic vascular resistance (SVR). SVR increases with peripheral vasoconstriction.

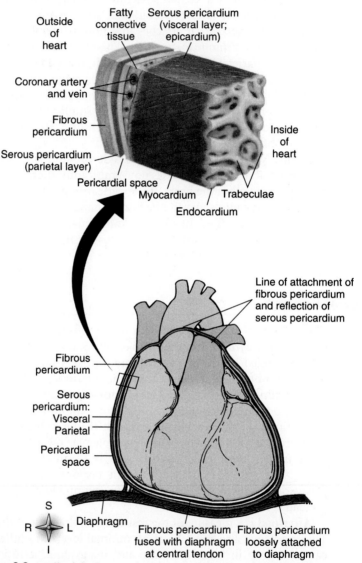

Figure 2-2. Wall of the heart. This section of the heart wall shows the fibrous pericardium, the parietal and visceral layers of the serous pericardium (with the pericardial space between them), the myocardium, and the endocardium. *(From Thibodeau GA, Patton KT:* Anatomy and physiology, *ed 5, St Louis, 2003, Mosby.)*

High afterload (increased PVR or SVR) caused by increased resistance to flow downstream from the heart leads to elevated back pressure on the pulmonic and aortic valves. For example, high PVR increases the pressure in the pulmonary artery and puts greater back pressure on the pulmonic valve during diastole when the valve is closing. This results in the pulmonic valve closing more loudly than normal (see Chapters 4 and 7).

The third factor that determines cardiac output is **contractility.** The heart must be healthy and well-nourished for optimal contractility. Poor contractility is common after a myocardial infarction, with diseases of the heart muscle (cardiomyopathies), and when electrolyte imbalances are present. Contractility is difficult to measure and usually is estimated by the simultaneous comparison of cardiac output, preload, and afterload. For example, if cardiac output is low and preload and afterload are normal, contractility is probably the problem. Contractility of the ventricles affects the force that closes the A-V valves. Increased contractility closes the valves forcefully, whereas decreased contractility closes them with less force.

One indicator of contractility is **ejection fraction.** This is the portion of the end-diastolic volume that is ejected out of the ventricle with each contraction. Normally the ejection fraction is about 0.65 to 0.70, or 65% to 70%. Heart disease that negatively affects contractility will cause the ejection fraction to fall.

☞ Key Point

Cardiac output is determined by how much blood fills the heart before contraction (preload), how much resistance there is to flow out of the heart (afterload), and the ability of the myocardium to contract (contractility).

HEART TOPOGRAPHY

The heart is located between the lungs in the mediastinum. It lies mostly to the left of the midsternal line and typically assumes an oblique position (Figure 2-3). The body build of the patient, chest configuration, condition of the lungs, and position of the diaphragm determine the exact position of the heart. Thus its position may vary from patient to patient. Typically, the heart lies obliquely in the chest of a person with an average build and normal chest configuration. The heart assumes a more vertical position in the tall, slender person and in those with a low, flat diaphragm, as in emphysema. The heart may shift

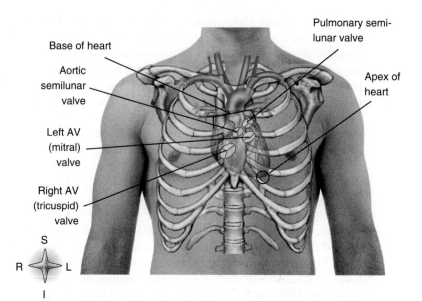

Figure 2-3. Topographic view of the heart. Note that the base of the heart is the upper portion and the apex is the lower portion. *(From Wilson SF, Giddens JF:* Health assessment for nursing practice, *ed 2, St Louis, 2001, Mosby. [As appears in Thibodeau GA, Patton KT:* Anatomy and physiology, *ed 5, St Louis, 2003, Mosby.])*

left or right when unilaterial lung disorders are present. For example, collapse (atelectasis) of the right lung will cause the heart to shift to the right, thus assuming a more central position. Tension pneumothorax or a large pleural effusion will push the heart toward the unaffected side. Atelectasis on one side will cause the heart to shift towards the atelectatic lung.

The upper portion of the heart is known as the *base* of the heart and consists primarily of the right and left atria. The base of the heart is located mostly under the center of the sternum; however, the right atrium may extend minimally to the right of the sternum (see Figure 2-3). The lower portion of the heart is known as the *apex,* which extends downward and to the patient's left to the fifth intercostal space at the left midclavicular line. The apex of the heart comprises the right and left ventricles. The right ventricle is located more anteriorly and lies directly under the lower portion of the sternum in healthy people. The left ventricle is located more posteriorly and lies beneath the ribs on the left extending away from the sternum.

Chapter Highlights

- The heart is a four-chamber organ that pumps blood. It is divided into the left and right sides, and each side has its own atrium and ventricle.
- The left side of the heart is a high-pressure system that pumps blood throughout the body.
- The right side of the heart is a low-pressure system that pumps blood to the lungs for oxygenation of the blood and elimination of carbon dioxide from the blood.
- The mitral (or bicuspid) valve is located between the left atrium and left ventricle. It closes during ventricular contraction and prevents the backflow of blood into the left atrium and pulmonary veins.
- The aortic valve is located at the opening of the aorta. It opens during systole and closes during diastole. It prevents the backflow of blood into the left ventricle.
- The tricuspid valve is located between the right atrium and the right ventricle. It closes during systole and prevents the backflow of blood into the right atrium and systemic venous system.
- The pulmonic valve is located at the opening of the pulmonary artery. It opens during systole and closes during diastole. It prevents the backflow of blood into the right ventricle.
- The four valves of the heart open and close normally in response to changes in pressure on one side of the valve as compared with the other side.
- The amount of blood pumped each minute by each ventricle is known as the *cardiac output.*
- Cardiac output is a function of how much blood fills the heart before systole (preload), how much resistance there is to flow out of the ventricles (afterload), and the contractility of the myocardium.
- The heart lies obliquely in the center of the chest with the lower portion (apex) extending down and to the patient's left. The upper portion of the heart (base) is primarily located under the center of the sternum.

Review Questions

1. Which chamber of the heart is most responsible for pumping oxygenated blood to all areas of the body to maintain tissue oxygenation?
   A. Right atrium
   B. Right ventricle
   C. Left atrium
   D. Left ventricle

2. What is the normal peak pressure in the right ventricle during systole?
   A. 25 mm Hg
   B. 50 mm Hg
   C. 120 mm Hg
   D. 150 mm Hg

Continued

Review Questions—cont'd

3. What is the normal peak pressure in the left ventricle during systole?
   A. 25 mm Hg
   B. 50 mm Hg
   C. 120 mm Hg
   D. 150 mm Hg

4. True or False
   Ventricular filling occurs during diastole.

5. True or False
   Stroke volume is the volume of blood ejected by the atrium with each contraction.

6. What valve is located between the right atrium and the right ventricle?
   A. Mitral valve
   B. Pulmonic valve
   C. Aortic valve
   D. Tricuspid valve

7. What valve is located between the left atrium and left ventricle?
   A. Mitral valve
   B. Pulmonic valve
   C. Aortic valve
   D. Tricuspid valve

8. Which of the following valves prevent regurgitation of blood back into the left ventricle during diastole?
   A. Mitral valve
   B. Pulmonic valve
   C. Aortic valve
   D. Tricuspid valve

9. True or False
   The heart valves are not influenced directly by the sympathetic nervous system.

10. True or False
    The pericardium normally provides lubrication to permit low-friction movement of the heart.

11. Which of the following is defined as the amount of ventricular filling during diastole?
    A. Preload
    B. Afterload
    C. Contractility
    D. Stroke volume

Review Questions—cont'd

12. Which of the following is a measure of resistance to flow out of the ventricle during systole?
- A. Preload
- B. Afterload
- C. Contractility
- D. Stroke volume

13. What is the normal ejection fraction of the left ventricle?
- A. 25%
- B. 40%
- C. 70%
- D. 90%

14. What portion of the heart is most anterior and lies directly under the lower portion of the sternum in the healthy adult?
- A. Left ventricle
- B. Right ventricle
- C. Base of the heart
- D. None of the above

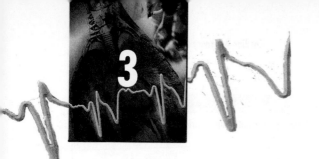

Fundamentals of Sound

Ernie Schwab, PhD

OBJECTIVES

After reading this chapter, you will be able to recognize and describe the following:
- The definition of sound.
- The characteristics of sound that can be measured.
- The factors that affect sound conduction.
- The factors that cause sound attenuation.

KEY TERMS

absorption	frequency	sound
acoustical impedance	Hertz	sound wave
amplitude	intensity	subsonic sound
attenuation	pitch	ultrasonic
compressional wave	reflection	sound

INTRODUCTION

The technique of chest auscultation is not very difficult to master. Understanding and interpreting the sounds that come from within the chest, however, is a greater challenge. An important topic that is often overlooked in the discussion of auscultation is the fundamentals of sound. The purpose of this chapter is to provide the reader with a basic understanding of sound physics as it relates to chest auscultation. Emphasis is placed on describing how sound is created, conducted, and measured. In addition, the variables that influence sound conduction and perception are presented. The reader is referred to the bibliography at the end of this chapter for more details on the physics of sound.

WHAT IS SOUND?

Sound is defined as the propagation of energy by a mechanical wave through matter. The source of sound creates a mechanical disturbance of some type before propagation through matter can occur. The mechanical disturbance can come from a large variety of sources, such as the striking of a bell, the turbulent airflow in the airways associated with breathing, or the sudden closure of heart valves. Once the energy of sound is generated, it is propagated (passed) from the source to the site of detection (most often the human ear) by setting into motion the molecules of the matter surrounding the sound source. For example, once a bell is struck, the walls vibrate rapidly and set into motion the molecules of air surrounding the bell (Figure 3-1).

As these vibrating molecules temporarily leave their own space, the density of air molecules in that space decreases. Simultaneously, the density of molecules in the adjacent space becomes momentarily greater (Figure 3-2). The zone of air in which molecular density has decreased is called a *zone of rarefaction*, whereas the adjacent zone of higher molecular density is a *zone of condensation*. The increase in molecular density at a zone of condensation produces a corresponding increase in air pressure within that zone. This transient increase in air pressure is referred to as a **compressional wave.**

Three important points must be made regarding any compressional wave. First, when air molecules are vibrating back and forth, they are not ultimately traveling great distances from their original locations. Instead, they vibrate (oscillate) about their original location in space; that is, they oscillate in place. When the molecules cease oscillating, they reoccupy their original equilibrium location in space. They have not

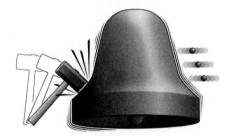

Figure 3-1. Illustration of sound-energy transfer from a sound source to surrounding air molecules. In this illustration, a bell is struck by a hammer, which makes the metal walls of the bell vibrate. That vibrational motion causes the walls of the bell to collide with adjacent air molecules, thus producing vibrational motion (oscillations) of those air molecules. As a result, kinetic energy from the hammer striking the bell is transferred to air molecules.

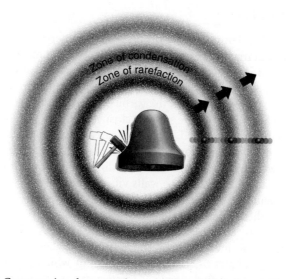

Figure 3-2. Compressional wave. When a bell is struck, adjacent air molecules are pushed a short distance from the bell, thus causing the space next to the bell to experience a lowered molecular density (zone of rarefaction). Simultaneously, a higher molecular density occurs within the region into which the original molecules were pushed (zone of condensation). As a result of molecular vibrations, these zones move outward as compressional waves (sound) in the direction indicated by the arrows.

been permanently displaced to some new location. Second, in a compressional wave, when oscillating molecules invade adjacent space and pressure in that space increases, collisions occur between the oscillating molecules and stationary molecules whose space the oscillating molecules have invaded. Thirdly, as a result of these collisions, energy is transferred from the oscillating molecules to the stationary molecules with which they collided, causing those stationary molecules to begin oscillating. The compressional wave moves out from its point of origin, inducing subsequent compressional waves in adjacent regions. This sequence of compressional waves continues over some time and distance, producing a *propagated compressional wave,* or **sound wave.** Notice that when a sound wave "carries" sound from a source to a destination, individual air molecules *do not* move the entire distance from the source to the destination. They simply oscillate in place, passing their kinetic energy to adjacent molecules, very much in a domino-like effect (Figure 3-3). Thus what is moved from source to destination is not the air molecules themselves but the kinetic energy of sound, an energy disturbance being passed from molecule to molecule until it is passed to the object of the destination (in our discussion, a human ear).

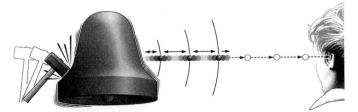

Figure 3-3. Sound wave. A sound wave is a propagated compressional wave. The illustration shows a compressional wave being propagated toward a listener. Propagation comprises a chain reaction of collisions between air molecules until the final molecules stimulate the hearing apparatus of the listener. Dark circles ● and solid arrows represent molecules already set in motion, while open circles ○ and dashed arrows represent stationary molecules that will ultimately be set in motion.

☞ Key Point

Sound is produced when a mechanical disturbance occurs and a compressional wave of energy spreads out from the source to the site of detection.

HOW IS SOUND MEASURED?

Sound waves, such as that depicted in Figure 3-2, are characterized by several important variables. The first is **frequency.** Sound wave frequency, measured in **Hertz** (Hz) or cycles per second, is a measure of the number of vibratory cycles completed in one second. As air molecules vibrate more rapidly, the number of vibratory cycles that occurs in 1 second increases, and sound frequency increases as a result. When the frequency of a sound wave increases, adjacent peaks (and troughs) move closer together. Conversely, decreasing sound frequency results in spreading peaks and troughs farther apart (Figure 3-4). *The human auditory system detects these changes in vibratory frequency as changes in the pitch of sound.* In summary, the objective measure of the number of sound vibrations per second is known as *frequency,* and the subjective perception by the human ear of the same quality is known as **pitch.**

The human ear is capable of detecting sound at *frequencies* between 20 Hz and 20,000 Hz. Sounds below 20 Hz are called **subsonic sounds;** those above 20,000 Hz are called **ultrasonic sounds.** Subsonic and ultrasonic sounds are undetectable by the human ear. Ultrasonic sound waves are used in medicine to image structures inside the body.

The power of sound is also measured and is a function of displacement. *Displacement* is a measure of the distance that a given molecule is moved from its equilibrium position during a vibratory cycle

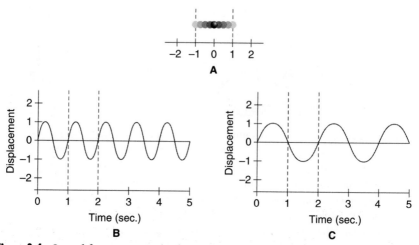

Figure 3-4. Sound frequency. **A,** A vibrating air molecule. Notice that when a sound wave causes air molecules to vibrate, vibration is longitudinal in a horizontal plane. The ruled axis represents relative units of displacement (distance the particle moves during vibration). This particle is being displaced 1 relative unit from its equilibrium position, in each direction. **B,** A plot of *displacement* vs. *time* for the vibrating particle from **A.** The molecule completes a vibration cycle once every millisecond (1000 Hertz sound). Displacement is 1 relative unit (as described in **A**). **C,** A plot of *displacement* vs. *time* for a molecule vibrating at half the frequency of the molecule in **B.** This molecule requires 2 milliseconds to complete one vibratory cycle (500 Hertz sound). The sound depicted by **B** is perceived as a higher pitch than the sound depicted by **C.**

(Figure 3-5). As a concept, displacement is particularly important because it is an indicator of the amount of energy invested in a given sound. Increasing the energy used to produce a sound wave results in a correlated increase in the displacement of molecules vibrating within the medium. Increasing particle displacement would be indicated in a compressional wave as a more dense zone of condensation. In a plot of displacement versus time, it appears as an increase in wave **amplitude**—that is, the perpendicular distance between an adjacent peak and trough is greater (see Figure 3-5). *Changes in wave amplitude are sensed as changes in sound **intensity** (loudness) by the human auditory system.*

Key Point

Objective measures of sound include frequency and amplitude. The subjective versions of these measurements are pitch and loudness, respectively.

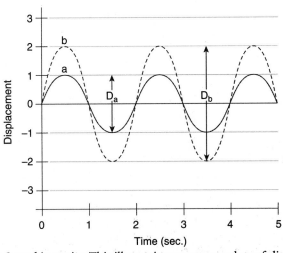

Figure 3-5. Sound intensity. This illustration represents plots of *displacement* vs. *time* for vibrating molecules from two different sound waves (wave *a* and wave *b*). Molecular displacement is greatest for wave *b* ($D_b > D_a$). Consequently, sound wave *b* is said to have a higher amplitude than wave *a*. Although both sound waves have the same pitch, sound wave *b* would be perceived as louder (a higher intensity sound) than sound wave *a*.

WHAT AFFECTS SOUND TRANSMISSION?

Sound can be conducted by any medium that has mass and elasticity. In general, that means sound can travel through anything except a vacuum. Because a perfect vacuum contains no molecules of any kind, the vibrations described earlier, necessary for production of compressional waves, cannot be produced; thus sound cannot occur.

The general rule for medium-specific efficiency and speed of sound wave conduction is this: *Increasing the density of a conducting medium increases both the efficiency and velocity of conduction.* We observed earlier in our discussion that a conducted sound wave consists of an energy disturbance that is passed sequentially from one molecule to the next. With that in mind, it should be intuitive that increasing the molecular density of a conducting medium will increase the number of molecular collisions per unit time while simultaneously decreasing the time lapse between collisions. Thus in a higher-density medium, an energy wave can travel more strongly and rapidly away from its source than is possible in a lower-density medium. In keeping with this general rule, Table 3-1 shows that at a given temperature, fluids conduct sounds better and faster than gases. Moreover, solids conduct sounds more effectively and at higher velocities than fluids.

Table 3-1	Speed of Sound in Different Media
Medium	Speed (m/sec)
Air	346
Fat	1450
Water	1495
Soft tissue	1540
Wood	3850
Bone	4080
Aluminum	5000
Steel	5200

Because the lungs have mass (e.g., cellular tissues, gases, fluids) and because they are elastic, sound can be conducted through the media that collectively comprise the lungs (see Chapter 1). Because the clinician is typically auscultating lung and heart sounds at the thoracic surface, the conducting media for those sounds include elements of the lung (for the lung sounds) and tissues that make up the thoracic wall (for lung and heart sounds). Sound waves travel less efficiently through the lungs because they are low-density structures normally. Changes increasing overall density (e.g., consolidation of the lungs as occurs with pneumonia) cause more efficient transmission of breath sounds and results in those sounds being louder over the affected region (see Chapter 6).

The temperature of the medium through which sound waves travel also plays a role in sound transmission. For each degree centigrade rise in temperature, the speed of sound increases by 61 cm/sec in air. The exact role of fever or hypothermia on the clinical interpretation of lung and heart sounds is not known; however, minor changes in body temperature probably does not influence interpretation.

Key Point

Sound waves travel faster and more efficiently through structures with greater density.

WHAT CAUSES ATTENUATION OF SOUND WAVES?

The energy of sound tends to decrease as it travels through time and space. This phenomenon is known as **attenuation.** Attenuation explains why it is more difficult to hear people speaking when they are farther away in comparison with when they are nearby. Likewise, it determines how effectively lung and heart sounds are conveyed to the body surface. Attenuation occurs as a result of three main factors: inverse square loss, reflection, and absorption. Each is explained in the following discussion.

Inverse Square Loss

The distance sound travels from its source to the point of detection has an especially strong effect on perceived sound intensity. Sound typically decays as a function of the inverse square of the distance traveled (this is known as *the Inverse Square Law*). This means that doubling the distance a sound travels will result in decreasing its intensity by a factor of four (Figure 3-6). Thus when one evaluates lung and heart sounds, auscultating closer to the sound source increases the intensity of that sound significantly (e.g., having the patient lean forward during cardiac auscultation allows easier detection of heart sounds because it causes the heart to be shifted toward the anterior chest wall).

Reflection and Absorption

In most natural situations, sound waves encounter obstacles to their propagation. When an obstacle lies in the path of a sound wave, it

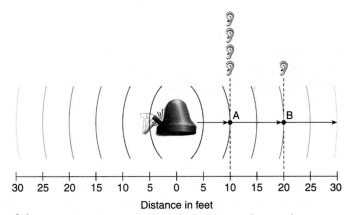

Figure 3-6. Inverse Square Law. When the bell is struck, sound waves move out from the bell in all directions, thus forming a series of concentric spheres (depicted here in two dimensions only). As sound travels farther from its source, it is increasingly attenuated (e.g., becomes quieter). For each doubling of distance, the sound is attenuated by a factor of four. Thus sound intensity 10 feet from the bell is four times greater than intensity 20 feet from the bell (the number of ears drawn above the axis indicate relative sound intensity at each location). Although this principle is depicted in one direction only in this figure, inverse square attenuation of sound occurs in every direction the sound wave is propagated.

disrupts transmission of that wave. Upon encountering the medium of which the obstacle is comprised, the sound wave will be impacted as follows. A portion of the sound wave will be **reflected** from the surface of the obstacle (e.g., fluid). That reflected portion will be propagated back through the original medium in which it was traveling. The remaining portion of the sound wave will enter the medium that presents the obstacle.

Some of that energy will be absorbed by the new medium. The amount of sound **absorption** is related to the density of the obstacle (thus bone is a much greater sound obstacle in comparison with the lung). The energy that is absorbed or reflected is lost to the process of sound transmission. The energy not absorbed or reflected will induce the molecules of the new medium to begin vibrating, and that sound will continue to be *transmitted* through the obstacle. However, the total energy of the sound wave will have been reduced as a result of loss to reflection and absorption (Figure 3-7).

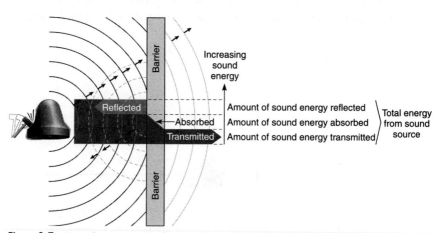

Figure 3-7. Sound attenuation due to change in conducting medium. When a sound wave encounters a change in the conducting medium (e.g., any sort of obstacle or change in density), it directly impacts the way the sound will continue to be propagated. If the density of the obstacle is greater than that of the original conducting medium, a portion of the sound will be reflected back in the original medium toward the sound source. The energy of the reflected wave is subtracted from the total energy of the propagated wave. Sound not reflected from the surface of the obstacle will be conducted into the medium of which the obstacle is comprised. That medium itself will absorb some of the sound energy. That absorbed sound energy is subtracted from the total energy of the propagated wave. Energy that remains after the energy losses caused by reflection and absorption comprises the sound energy transmitted when the propagated wave emerges from the obstacle.

In just such a way, sound in one room can be heard in an adjoining room because it is able to be propagated through the separating walls, although the intensity of the sound in the adjoining room is attenuated because of the processes of reflection and absorption as described previously. Similarly, when sounds generated in the interior of the lungs or heart are propagated toward the body surface, the transmission pathway is characterized by many inconsistencies in the conducting medium. These inconsistencies are responsible for a great deal of reflection and absorption of sound energy as transmission occurs toward the body surface.

Thus lung and heart sounds are subject to the modulations produced when a medium with a different characteristic impedance is encountered by the propagated wave. When pathologic changes occur within a lung (e.g., pneumonia) or chest wall (e.g., pleural effusion), those changes modify the characteristic impedance of at least a portion of the pathway. Resulting changes in the lung or heart sounds are identifiable and are described in Chapters 6 and 7.

Absorption of sound waves is also a function of sound frequency. The higher the frequency, the more rapidly the molecules of the conduction medium must move and the greater the energy expended in overcoming friction. For example, absorption of sounds at 10 M Hz (megahertz) by the body tissues is 10 times greater than sounds at 1 M Hz. Thus lower-frequency sounds are propagated through tissues (e.g., lung or chest wall) significantly better than higher frequency sounds because higher frequency sounds are more subject to attenuation due to absorption. This might explain why breath sounds heard over the lung are primarily heard as low-pitched sounds even though the source of the sound is high-pitched (see Chapter 6).

☞ Key Point

Attenuation of sound waves is a result of inverse square loss (distance), reflection, and absorption. Fluid reflects sound waves, whereas bone absorbs sound waves.

WHAT IS THE CAUSE OF SOUND REFLECTION?

When sound is conducted through a medium, various properties of the medium tend to impede its vibratory motion and thus sound transmission. The most important property in this regard is molecular density. As was discussed in the previous section, molecular density impacts the speed at which a sound wave is transmitted through a given medium. The mathematical product of a conducting medium's density and the speed of sound in that medium is defined to be the *characteristic imped-ance or* **acoustical impedance** of the medium.

Every medium has a unique characteristic impedance, determined as stated previously by the product of its density and sound transmitting velocity. When a sound wave is conducted exclusively through a single medium, without crossing the interface(s) between media, the degree to which the sound intensity is attenuated is a strict function of the Inverse Square Law. As a result, the efficiency of sound transmission is always highest when media boundaries are not crossed by sound waves. This rather ideal situation only occurs when a propagated wave is not obstructed by obstacles. But it was noted earlier that in most natural situations, sound waves *do* encounter obstacles to their propagation. This is certainly true of heart and lung sounds. Whenever the sound waves attempt to pass from tissue of one acoustical imped-ance value to one of significantly different acoustical impedance characteristics (e.g., lung to bone or lung to fluid), the intensity of the propagated wave will be reduced, primarily because of reflection. Thus listening to lung or heart sounds directly over ribs or the sternum is not useful. Likewise a large pleural effusion will result in reduced or absent breath sounds.

In general, when pathologic changes occur within a lung or chest wall, those changes modify the characteristic impedance of at least a portion of the pathway. Resulting changes in the lung or heart sounds are identifiable and are described in Chapters 6 and 7.

☞ Key Point

The interface between two structures of significantly different acoustical con-duction abilities will hinder sound wave propagation because of reflection.

Chapter Highlights

- Sound is defined as the propagation of energy by a mechanical wave through matter.
- Sound is propagated by the vibration of the molecules through which the mechanical wave is passing. The vibration of medium molecules creates a compressional wave (sound wave).
- Two important measures of sound are frequency (the number of vibrations per second) and amplitude (the power/velocity of the sound wave). Subjective indicators of these measurements are pitch and loudness, respectively.
- The most important factor that determines the speed of sound conductance is the density of the medium. Structures with greater density conduct sound at higher speed and with greater efficiency. Structures with a low density do not conduct sound waves effectively.

- The ability to hear sounds at a fixed distance from the sound source is inversely related to the distance between the site of sound production and the site of sound detection.
- Attenuation is the decrease in sound as it travels through time and space. The three primary factors that determine attenuation in the body are inverse square loss, absorption, and reflection. Obstacles to sound conduction cause the sound waves to be absorbed or reflected back toward the sound source. In either case, sound detection distal to the obstacle is impeded.
- Reflection of sound waves also occurs when they attempt to pass across tissues of significantly different acoustical impedance characteristics (e.g., air to bone or vice versa).

BIBLIOGRAPHY

- Berg RE, Stork DG: *The physics of sound*, ed 2, Englewood Cliffs, N.J., 1994, Prentice-Hall.
- Blauert J: *Spatial hearing: the psychophysics of human sound localization*, revised edition, Cambridge, Mass., 1996, MIT Press.
- Fleischer AC, Romero R, Manning FA et al: The principles and practice of ultrasonography, ed 4, Norwalk, Conn., 1991, Appleton and Lange.
- Pickles JO: *An introduction to the physiology of hearing*, ed 2, New York, 1992, Academic Press.
- Rossing TD, Moore FR, Wheeler PA: *The science of sound*, ed 3, San Francisco, 2001, Addison Wesley.
- Trinklein F: *Modern physics*, Austin, Tex., 1992, Holt, Rinehart and Winston, Inc.
- Yost WA: *Fundamentals of hearing*, ed 4, New York, 2000, Academic Press.
- Zwicker E, Fastl H, Frater H: *Psychoacoustics: facts and models*, ed 2, New York, 1999, Springer Verlag.

Review Questions

1. True or False

The density of air molecules in a zone of rarefaction is higher than the molecular density in an adjacent zone of condensation.

2. True or False

Sound is a propagated wave of increased pressure that moves directionally away from the source of sound.

3. True or False

High frequency sound has a lower pitch than low frequency sound.

4. True or False

Increasing the power in a sound wave increases the displacement of individual oscillating molecules.

Continued

Review Questions — cont'd

5. True or False

Sound can move only through gases, such as air; it cannot be propagated through solid or liquid media.

6. True or False

A conducting medium *can* absorb some of the energy of a propagated sound wave, thus reducing the final energy of the transmitted sound.

7. True or False

When a sound wave encounters an obstacle that is denser than the medium in which that sound is being conducted, at least part of the sound energy will be reflected from the surface of the obstacle.

8. True or False

Sound waves travel more efficiently through a hyperinflated lung than through a healthy lung.

9. True or False

When one is listening to lung sounds, the sounds should be loudest when auscultation is performed closest to the source of the sound.

10. True or False

Pathological changes in the lung that result in changes in tissue density should not have any effect on auscultated lung sounds.

11. When a bell is struck, the molecules of air adjacent to the bell are set into vibratory motion, and the sound wave produced causes the vibrating air molecules to:
   A. Move the entire distance to the point of sound detection
   B. Move a distance equal to the inverse of the square of the entire distance to the point of sound detection
   C. Oscillate in place
   D. None of the above is correct

12. The velocity of sound conduction is usually greatest in:
   A. Liquids
   B. Solids
   C. Gases
   D. A vacuum

13. A sound wave generated from airways might encounter which of the following as it propagates outward?
   A. Fluid
   B. Soft connective tissue
   C. Dense osseous material
   D. All of the above are correct

Review Questions—cont'd

14. When a sound is produced within a lung, which part of that sound is most likely to be perceived at the body surface?
    A. Most of the reflected sound
    B. Absorbed sound
    C. Attenuated sound
    D. None of the above can be perceived at the body surface

15. Loud, high-pitched sound would be characterized by which type of measurement?
    A. Low amplitude, low frequency
    B. Low amplitude, high frequency
    C. High amplitude, low frequency
    D. High amplitude, high frequency

Bedside Patient Assessment

OBJECTIVES

After reading this chapter, you will be able to recognize and describe the following:

- Useful techniques for interviewing the patient with cardiac or pulmonary symptoms.
- The common symptoms of cardiopulmonary disease and the significant characteristics of each to identify in the interview.
- Correct techniques for inspection, palpation, percussion, and auscultation of the chest.
- The common clinical signs associated with cardiopulmonary disease and the significance of each finding.

KEY TERMS

apical impulse	heave	pectus carinatum
barrel chest	hemoptysis	pectus excavatum
bulging	hepatomegaly	personal space
clubbing	intimate space	platypnea
copious	jugular venous	point of maximum
cor pulmonale	distension (JVD)	impulse (PMI)
costochondritis	lift	precordium
cough	lymphadenopathy	purulent
crepitation	orthopnea	retraction
cyanosis	paradoxical pulse	social space
dyspnea	paroxysmal nocturnal	stethoscope
fremitus	dyspnea	thrills

Patient assessment is done for two primary reasons: to diagnose the patient's problem and to monitor his or her response to therapy. A large variety of procedures and tests are available to clinicians who are performing patient assessments; however, none is more important than the bedside assessment. Bedside assessment is defined as the combination of interviewing and physical examination of the patient. It is often the first interaction between the patient and the health care provider, and when done correctly, it provides valuable information that cannot be obtained in any other way.

The purpose of this chapter is to describe the techniques of interviewing and physical examination of the patient. Emphasis is placed on the use of these techniques in patients with cardiopulmonary disease. In addition, emphasis is placed on the technique of chest auscultation for normal and abnormal lung and heart sounds.

THE MEDICAL HISTORY

The medical history is an account of the events in the patient's life that have relevance to his or her physical and mental health. The role of each health care provider varies somewhat with regard to the medical history. For example, the attending physician has the responsibility of completing a thorough interview to obtain information about the patient's current and past medical problems. Other health care providers may interview the patient more briefly to identify current problems and changes in those problems as treatment is rendered. Regardless of your exact role, you must be able to communicate with the patient to obtain answers to medical questions and review the patient's chart to identify key information about his or her past medical history. For these reasons, this chapter will address two important issues: how to conduct an interview and how to review the medical chart.

Fundamentals of Interviewing

Interviewing and patient assessment require the examiner to develop an appropriate bedside manner. One important aspect of developing an appropriate bedside manner is the proper use of space around the patient. Begin your encounter with new patients by introducing yourself in the **social space** (4 to 10 feet from the patient). After introducing yourself and a brief period of conversation, it is now appropriate to move to the **personal space** (2 to 4 feet from the patient) (Figure 4-1). The interview is conducted in the personal space, which allows for quiet conversation with the patient and allows him or her to answer personal questions without having to respond so loudly that others not involved in the interview could hear the answers easily.

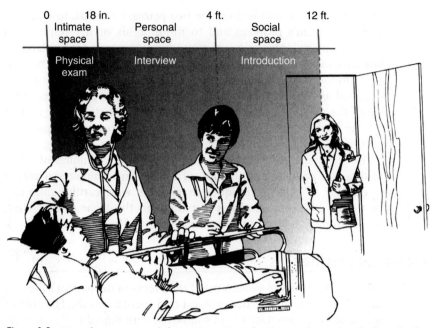

Figure 4-1. Use of space around the patient. Introduction to the patient is done in the social space (4 to 10 feet), interviewing in the pers3p6.357onal space (2 to 4 feet), and physical examination in the intimate space (0 to 2 feet). *(From Wilkins RL, Krider SJ, Sheldon RL: Clinical assessment in respiratory care, ed 4, St Louis, 2000, Mosby.)*

Physical examination is done in the **intimate space** (up to 18 inches) and should be entered only after you have introduced yourself in the social space and interviewed the patient in the personal space in most cases. Exceptions occur such as when the patient is in urgent need of treatment. In such cases, entering the intimate space more rapidly is acceptable. It is inappropriate to interview the patient in the intimate space.

Begin the interview session by making the environment comfortable for the patient. This may call for pulling the curtain to provide privacy or waiting to do the interview until the bathroom has been visited. Next, move to a position that conveys interest and a relaxed atmosphere. This requires you to face the patient and sit at a level equal to the patient. Standing over the patient conveys superiority and may prevent him or her from communicating openly.

The fundamental principles of interviewing the pulmonary patient are the same as for any patient. These principles include careful listening and questioning in association with skillful observation. The initial and subsequent interviews usually center around a discussion of the patient's chief complaints or symptoms. Each complaint should be probed to identify all important details such as when it started, what seemed to provoke it, how severe it is, what seems to make it better (if anything), has it ever happened before, and the use of any medications used to treat it. Once the initial interview is completed, subsequent interviews should focus on any changes in the symptoms that may have occurred with treatment or simply with the passing of time.

An important aspect of any interview is the use of eye contact. Little or no eye contact implies a lack of genuine interest in the patient and is a common error among novice interviewers. A general rule of thumb is to look at the patient whenever he or she is speaking except when you are taking notes. It is also a good idea to look at the patient when you are asking questions; this allows you to see evidence of confusion, pain, sorrow, etc. This may allow you to use an appropriate follow-up question or signal when to clarify the previous question.

The more common symptoms seen in patients with cardiopulmonary disease are discussed in the following pages. This knowledge is helpful to the interviewer beacause it provides the framework for important questions to ask during the interview.

☞ Key Point

Interviewing is done in the personal space (2 to 4 feet from the patient). This space should be entered only after you have established a rapport with the patient in the social space (4 to 10 feet from the patient).

Cough

Cough is required for self-cleansing of the airways but may be secondary to inflammation or irritation of the airway lining. This symptom readily brings attention to the lungs. An acute cough is difficult for the patient to ignore in contrast to a chronic cough, which the patient may feel is customary or habitual. This is particularly true of the smoker's cough. The typical smoker often has a daily ritual of morning cigarette, newspaper, coffee, and 3 or 4 minutes of productive coughing. When interviewed, however, the smoker often denies having a problem with chronic cough. The patient's spouse may be helpful in such cases.

Other factors to be considered in addition to the acuteness or chronicity of the cough are the circumstances of the cough: Does the cough only occur with laughing, exercise, weather changes, or exposure to suspected allergenic materials? This type of coughing might occur in a patient with reversible bronchospasm or asthma. Coughing with a change in body position may suggest chronic bronchitis or bronchogenic carcinoma.

Table 4-1	Types and Causes of Cough	
Description	Possible causes
Weak	Neuromuscular disease, emphysema, pain from abdominal or thoracic surgery
Dry, acute	Viral respiratory infection, gastroesophageal reflux, exposure to second-hand smoke, airway tumor
Dry, chronic	Pulmonary fibrosis, nervous habit, postnasal drip
Loose, acute	Pulmonary infection
Loose, chronic	Chronic bronchitis, cystic fibrosis, bronchiectasis, asthma
Paroxysmal nocturnal	Left heart failure, asthma, gastroesophageal reflux disease (GERD)
Brassy or hoarse	Laryngitis, croup, laryngeal tumor, aortic aneurysm

The character of the cough (whether it is dry or productive) is also of importance. A dry cough—often described as barking (seal-like), brassy, or hoarse—usually indicates an acute irritative or inflammatory process that involves the pharynx or larynx. A cough with this description could be caused by the inhalation of noxious fumes or by an allergy leading to an irritated hypopharynx and postnasal drip. Most likely, however, a simple viral or atypical bacterial infection is the cause. A neoplasm (abnormal formation of tissue) in the respiratory tree, benign or malignant, would lead to coughing by direct mechanical irritation of the respiratory tissues, thus resulting in cough-receptor stimulation. Aspiration of foreign material will cause acute episodes of coughing. A dry, nonproductive cough is also seen in some patients with pulmonary fibrosis. See Table 4-1 for a description of the terms used to describe coughing and their possible significance.

A productive cough produces pulmonary secretions; it is commonly seen with acute bacterial infections that affect the airways and with diseases of the airways such as bronchitis. A productive cough that persists for months or years, often worse in the morning, suggests chronic bronchitis. In fact, the diagnosis of chronic bronchitis is made on the basis of the patient who has a productive cough for at least 3 months of the year for 2 consecutive years (assuming no other disease, such as tuberculosis, explains the cough). Commonly, the cough is associated with a smoking history. Bronchiectasis, an insidious disease characterized by permanent dilation of the bronchial tubes, also is associated with chronic cough and sputum production. Often a profuse amount of secretions (e.g., 2 to 3 cupfuls of phlegm), termed **copious,** is produced each day by the patient with bronchiectasis.

Sputum with an acute productive cough may be **purulent** (containing pus) or non-purulent (i.e., the silicone-like plugs produced by the typical asthmatic patient) (Table 4-2). An acutely purulent sputum

Table 4-2	Terms Associated with the Description of Sputum	
Term	Meaning	Possible causes
Mucoid	Clear, thick	Airways disease such as asthma
Purulent	Pus-containing	Airway or lung infection
Copious	Large amounts	Bronchiectasis
Fetid	Foul smelling	Infection, lung abcess, bronchiectasis

suggests infection; the sample should be gram stained and analyzed under the microscope for the presence of pus cells and bacteria. A concentration of greater than 25 leukocytes per high power field (hpf) suggests infection. The visualization of many epithelial cells under hpf highly suggests oral contamination. The gram stain obtained in this situation could be unreliable because the analyzed sample may represent oral rather than lung pathogens.

Other important information obtained by a reliable gram stain includes the presence of fungi as well as the size and shape of the bacteria. A wet-mount preparation or Wright stain to differentiate between the presence of eosinophils and neutrophils can be helpful in determining whether the cough is caused by an allergic disorder or infection. Numerous eosinophils in a sputum specimen can indicate an allergic response, parasitic infestation, or other serious pulmonary disorder, whereas an increase in neutrophils is common with an infectious process.

Dyspnea

Dyspnea, or literally "difficult breathing," is a symptom that is likely to be reported by the patient as "smothering" or a "tightness in the chest." Patients with dyspnea may also report that they are "quickly out of breath" or that they "can't take a deep breath." Occasionally, the patient may appear to be short of breath but will not complain of difficult breathing when asked. Dyspnea can be classified as occurring "while at rest," "with exertion only," "while lying down" (**orthopnea),** or "upon awakening at night" (**paroxysmal nocturnal dyspnea).** Dyspnea that is present only in the upright position is known as **platypnea.**

The etiology of dyspnea is potentially far reaching; it ranges from physiologic dyspnea (that associated with physical exertion) to the dyspnea of cardiac failure (as output from the left ventricle fails to keep up with metabolic needs). Dyspnea may also be psychogenic, as when associated with hysterical hyperventilation.

In patients with lung disease, dyspnea usually is caused by a disorder that results in an increased work of breathing, such as restrictive defects that decrease the compliance of the lungs or chest wall, or obstructive defects with partial airway obstruction (Table 4-3).

Table 4-3 | Causes of Dyspnea

General category	Examples
Increased WOB due to obstruction of the airways	Asthma, COPD, cystic fibrosis
Increased WOB due to low lung compliance	Pneumonia, ARDS, pulmonary edema, pulmonary fibrosis
Increased WOB due to chest wall abnormalities	Kyphoscoliosis, obesity, broken ribs
Increases in the drive to breathe	Hypoxemia, hypercarbia, acidosis

Restrictive lung disease can lead to intense dyspnea, especially with exertion. Obstructive defects lead to dyspnea as a result of the increased resistance to air movement through the airways. This increases the work of breathing and causes the patient to feel dyspneic. Factors that increase the drive to breathe (e.g., hypoxemia, acidosis) contribute to the sensation of dyspnea in patients with an increase in the work of breathing.

In patients with heart disease, dyspnea occurs with exertion when cardiac output fails to meet oxygen demands of skeletal muscles. This is common with mitral or aortic valve disease, with cardiomyopathies, and after myocardial infarction that damages the left ventricle. Differentiating patients with dyspnea due to heart disease from those with dyspnea due to lung disease can be a challenge that requires careful interviewing, physical examination, and selected laboratory tests.

The degree of dyspnea present should be quantified in some patients, especially when the patient suffers from chronic shortness of breath. Documenting the patient's perception of the severity of the dyspnea can be helpful in determining how sick the patient is and the effectiveness of therapy. The degree of dyspnea present can be assessed by asking the patient how far he or she can walk on a flat surface at a normal pace before stopping to rest. Clinicians also can use simple documentation forms that call for the patient to rate the degree of dyspnea present by circling a number from 1 to 10, with 1 indicating little or no dyspnea and 10 being the most severe case (a scale commonly referred to as the Borg Scale). Measures of the degree of dyspnea present may correlate poorly with objective parameters such as peak flow and PaO_2 but remain important in evaluating the patient's comfort level and general quality of life.

✍ Key Point

Dyspnea occurs when the work of breathing is high and intensifies if the drive to breathe is increased.

Hemoptysis

Hemoptysis (coughing up blood) is particularly alarming to the individual who experiences it. Usually the complaint is "blood-tinged sputum." Although chronic bronchitis is commonly a cause of hemoptysis, this symptom should never be ignored because serious lung or cardiac disorders (e.g., bronchogenic cancer, tuberculosis, pulmonary embolism, and mitral stenosis) can also cause it. Determining whether the lungs actually are the source of the blood reported is also important (Table 4-4). A trivial nosebleed or serious esophageal variceal bleeding may be erroneously reported as hemoptysis. Hemoptysis is benign in most cases, especially in the patient with a negative smoking history. Although rare, the amount of hemoptysis can be enough to be life threatening.

Chest Pain

Chest pain is most often considered the cardinal symptom of cardiac disease but may be the result of pulmonary disease as well. Most often, chest pain originates from the muscles, ligaments, ribs, or costochondral junctions in the chest wall/rib cage. Usually chest pain associated with pulmonary disease is caused by the stimulation of pain fibers in the chest wall and/or parietal pleura. Pleuritic chest pain is located laterally and is associated with an inflamed parietal pleura. This pain is predominantly present during inspiration and is described as sharp and severe. Patients usually notice that the pain is lessened by lying on the affected side, which decreases movement of that side of the chest (autosplinting). This sign usually indicates involvement of the parietal pleura by such diseases as tuberculosis, pulmonary infarction, pneumonia, spontaneous pneumothorax, or cancer.

Nonpleuritic chest pain is a problem in many patients with heart disease. This type of pain, commonly called *angina pectoris,* is located centrally in the chest and is not altered by changes in breathing pattern. The patient often describes the pain as pressure on his or her sternum or as a squeezing feeling that sometimes radiates to the shoulder, arm, or jaw. In patients that suffer a myocardial infarction ("heart attack"),

Table 4-4	Distinguishing Characteristics of Hemoptysis versus Hematemasis	
	Hemoptysis	*Hematemasis*
History	Lung disease	Gastrointestinal disease
Patient statement	Coughed from lung	Vomited from stomach
Color	Bright red	Dark red
pH	High (alkaline)	Low (acidic)
Associated symptoms	Dyspnea, cough	Nausea, stomach pain

the chest discomfort is sometimes described as "feels like an elephant is sitting on my chest". Patients with cardiac chest pain often have a history of heart disease. This type of pain must be rapidly identified because prompt and proper treatment is essential. Esophagitis from reflux of gastric contents is a common cause of chest pain. Often called *heartburn,* this pain is commonly substernal in location and is quickly relieved by antacids.

Airway inflammation may lead to a pain described as a burning sensation and usually is pinpointed as retrosternal. Tracheal irritation as a result of viral tracheitis, exposure to extreme cold, or inhalation of noxious fumes can lead to pain of this type.

☞ Key Point

Chest pain that is located laterally and increases with breathing is likely to be caused by pleural inflammation.

Fever

Fever is present when the patient's body temperature elevates because of disease. Patients with viral or bacterial respiratory infections usually have a fever. Tuberculosis, pulmonary embolism, pneumonia, and fungal infection are possible sources of fever in patients with respiratory symptoms.

Fever is often the result of excessive heat production in the body when phagocytosis is occurring or when the hypothalamic set point is increased in response to disease. Elevation of body temperature causes the oxygen consumption and carbon dioxide production to increase. The patient with significant fever will breathe at a more rapid rate to accommodate the increase in metabolism. A fever that results from bacterial infections is commonly accompanied by shaking chills.

Reviewing the Patient's Documented Medical History

The major categories of the medical history are presented in Box 4-1. The most important sections to review are the history of present illness (HPI) and the past medical history (PMH). The HPI typically describes the current medical problems and the circumstances surrounding each problem. For example, if the patient had a recent onset of chest pain, the HPI should describe when it started, how severe it was and is, what made it worse or better, and various other details that may be important. The past medical history describes important medical problems the patient has had in the past. For example, if the patient has a history of asthma, COPD, heart disease, cancer, or stroke, it will be reported here in the PMH. Other categories of the typical medical history are presented in the following discussion.

Box 4-1	CATEGORIES OF THE MEDICAL HISTORY

Patient identification
Chief complaints
History of present illness
Past medical history
Family history
Occupational history
Smoking history
Review of systems

☞ **Key Point**

The HPI describes the details surrounding each symptom and should be familiar to any person providing care to the patient.

Review of Systems

The review of systems is necessary to determine whether the disease is confined to the cardiopulmonary system or whether the cardiac or pulmonary complaints are a manifestation of illness elsewhere (e.g., conjunctivitis and rhinitis in asthma, sinusitis in bronchiectasis, joint pains, alopecia, depigmentation, and erythema nodosum in sarcoidosis). Aspiration of postnasal drainage secretions or refluxed gastric contents into the airways at night can cause or exacerbate chronic bronchitis and asthma. If this is overlooked initially as the cause, the airway problem is difficult to control.

Occupational History

The patient's occupational history is often very important. Has the patient been in contact with coal, asbestos, or silica? The dust of these inorganic materials can lodge in the airways and lungs, thus causing significant disease over time. Other occupational exposures could include molds, pigeons, solvents, paints, etc. Geographical history must include travel, immigration, and region of permanent residence. This is especially important if one suspects diseases such as coccidioidomycosis, tuberculosis, or histoplasmosis.

Smoking History

Tobacco smoke inhalation, either primary or secondary, is clearly the leading cause of respiratory disease in adults. Lung cancer, heart disease, stroke, and chronic obstructive pulmonary disease are linked directly to cigarette consumption. The number of cigarettes smoked usually is recorded by "pack years." This is determined by multiplying the average number of packs smoked daily by the years smoked. For example, if a patient has smoked about 2 packs/day for the past 20 years, he or she has a 40 pack/year smoking history. The more "pack years" smoked, the greater is the risk of disease. The interview should identify when the patient started smoking and any attempts to quit. Exposure to second-hand smoke is associated also with an increased risk of cardiopulmonary disease.

Family and Social History

The family history includes any history of asthma, hayfever, eczema, premature emphysema, chronic bronchitis, cardiac disease, and cystic fibrosis in other family members. The social history may identify the excessive use of alcohol or abuse of other substances. Alcoholism can be associated with periods of loss of consciousness (as in binge drinkers), a decreased efficiency of lung defense mechanisms, and a consequent predisposition to aspiration pneumonia as well as bacterial pneumonias of the usual type. Chronic abuse of alcohol is also associated with cardiomyopathy.

Pharmacologic History

Determining the medications the patient is taking is crucial to the initial assessment. Sometimes the medication regimen is not optimal (i.e., important medications that might be helpful are missing) and sometimes the patient is on medications that may cause respiratory problems (i.e., angiotensin converting enzyme [ACE] inhibitor–induced cough and beta blocker–induced bronchospasm). Family members may be helpful in identifying the names of all medications the patient is taking.

PHYSICAL EXAMINATION

The initial physical examination is done by the attending physician to identify all abnormalities and further clarify the cause of the patient's symptoms. Subsequent examinations are done by other health care providers to assess the patient's response to treatment and monitor his or her overall well-being. Physical examination skills are not difficult to learn but require repeated practice to master. The time-honored combination of inspection, palpation, percussion for resonance, and auscultation are the major components of each examination. How these components are applied to assess the pulmonary system will be presented first. This is followed by a description of the cardiac examination.

Chest Inspection—Lungs

Mastery of the art of inspection may take a little time but can be very fruitful, especially if the examiner has a thorough knowledge of the

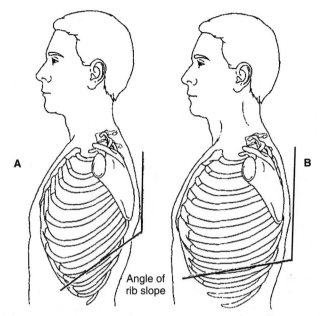

Angle of
rib slope

Figure 4-2. **A,** Normal chest configuration; **B,** increased AP diameter with hypertrophy of the sternocleidomastoid muscle in the neck, typical of patients with chronic obstructive lung disease. *(From Barkauskas VH, Baumann LC, Darling-Fisher CS:* Health and physical assessment, *ed 3, St Louis, 2002, Mosby.)*

topographic anatomy (see Chapter 1) and is comfortable and not hurried. A well-lit, warm room is essential for proper inspection. Place the patient in the sitting position stripped to the waist. For female patients, always prevent embarrassing exposure with adequate draping.

Note whether the patient is in pain and whether the respirations are noisy or distressed. Identify whether the patient is using accessory muscles to breathe. Use of the accessory muscles implies that the work of breathing is increased, as with airways obstruction or reduced lung compliance. Pay careful attention to the skin and nutritional state. Some chronic lung diseases result in poor eating habits and malnutrition. Observe the patient for localized areas of **bulging** or **retraction** and for the presence of thoracic deformities, such as an increase in anteroposterior diameter (**"barrel chest"**). This is classic in the patient with emphysema (Figure 4-2).

Other thoracic deformities of note include **pectus carinatum** (pigeon breast), characterized by the upper ribs bending inward and thrusting the sternum outwards like the keel of a ship (Figure 4-3). The "funnel breast" of **pectus excavatum** (the reverse of carinatum), when severe, can diminish vital capacity; however, it is usually a mild, asymptomatic, congenital defect of cosmetic concern only. The examiner

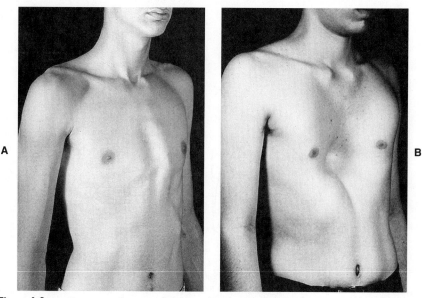

Figure 4-3. **A,** Pectus carinatum (pigeon chest). **B,** Pectus excavatum (funnel chest). Deformities of the thorax. *(From Seidel HM, Ball JW, Dains JE, et al:* Mosby's guide to physical examination, *ed 5, St Louis, 2003, Mosby.)*

should pay special attention to an exaggerated thoracic and lumbar spinal curvature (kyphosis and scoliosis) because these findings may limit lung expansion, thus causing a significant restrictive defect.

The patient's breathing pattern can provide useful clues as to the condition of the respiratory system. Patients breathing at a normal rate (<18/min) with minimal effort rarely have significant respiratory disease. Rapid and shallow breathing often is associated with significant loss of lung volume (restrictive disease). Atelectasis, pulmonary edema, and pneumonia are common examples. The greater the reduction in lung volume, the more the respiratory rate increases. Obstructive lung disease is characterized by deeper breaths, with the patient inhaling rapidly but exhaling slowly. The prolonged expiratory time seen obstructive lung disease occurs as the intrathoracic airways narrow on exhalation, thus making it difficult to deflate the lung. A prolonged inspiratory time indicates upper airway obstruction (e.g., croup or epiglottitis).

Other areas of the body should be carefully inspected. The digits are inspected for **clubbing** (abnormal enlargement of the distal phalanges) (Figure 4-4). Clubbing is a nonspecific finding often associated with lung cancer and some chronic cardiac disorders (e.g., congenital cyanotic heart disease). The exact mechanism for it remains unknown.

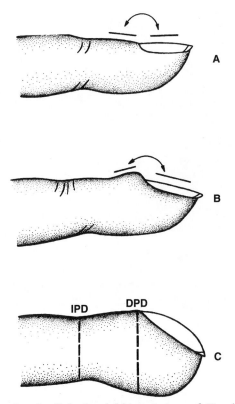

Figure 4-4. Assessing the digits for clubbing; **A,** normal; **B,** mild clubbing; **C,** severe clubbing. *(From Wilkins RL, Krider SJ, Sheldon RL:* Clinical assessment in respiratory care, *ed 4, St Louis, 2000, Mosby.)*

The neck is inspected for the presence of **jugular venous distension (JVD)** (Figure 4-5). JVD occurs with right heart failure when pulmonary vascular resistance is elevated chronically. This is common in patients with chronic lung disease that causes hypoxemia. It also occurs as a result of right heart failure subsequent to left heart failure. When right heart failure occurs as a result of lung disease, it is called **cor pulmonale.** JVD may be difficult to appreciate in patients with a short, muscular neck.

The presence or lack of cyanosis must be documented during physical examination. **Cyanosis** is a bluish discoloration of the skin or mucous membranes due to the presence of unsaturated hemoglobin. Peripheral cyanosis is present when the patient's digits and other peripheral regions are blue. Peripheral cyanosis indicates that circulation is not optimal and is often associated with cool/cold hands and feet. Central cyanosis is present when the patient has bluish discoloration of the oral mucosa

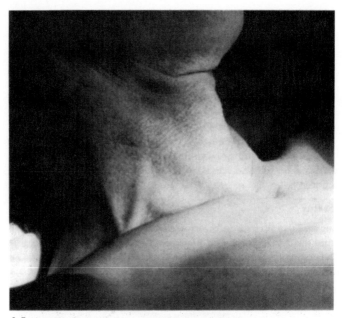

Figure 4-5. Jugular venous distention. *(From Daily EK, Schroeder JS: Techniques in bedside hemodynamic monitoring, ed 5, St Louis, 1994, Mosby.)*

and tongue. It is a sign of respiratory or cardiac failure with inadequate oxygen levels in the arterial blood. The patient's hemoglobin level affects the ability to detect cyanosis. Anemic patients will not demonstrate cyanosis until hypoxemia is severe; the patient with polycythemia will demonstrate cyanosis with mild to moderate hypoxemia.

☞ Key Point

The patient's breathing pattern is a reliable indicator of the underlying lung condition. Normal breathing essentially rules out serious lung disease. Rapid and shallow breathing suggests a loss of lung volume. A prolonged expiratory time indicates airways obstruction.

Chest Auscultation—Lungs

Auscultation, which is the act of listening to sounds produced in the body, has no peer in the evaluation of the state of bronchial patency and the assessment of normal and abnormal breath sounds. It is performed best with the aid of a **stethoscope.** The basic stethoscope does not

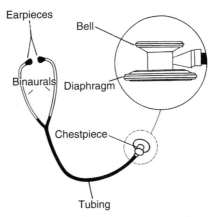

Figure 4-6. Acoustic stethoscope. *(From Wilkins RL, Krider SJ, Sheldon RL: Clinical assessment in respiratory care, ed 4, St Louis, 2000, Mosby.)*

amplify sound but assists in filtering out extraneous noises. Most modern stethoscopes consist of a bell, diaphragm, tubing, and earpieces (Figure 4-6). The diaphragm chestpiece is more receptive to high-pitched sounds, whereas the bell is best for evaluating low-pitched sounds (such as certain heart sounds). The diaphragm is usually better for evaluating normal and abnormal lung sounds. Chapter 5 describes the history of the stethoscope.

With the patient in a quiet room, apply the diaphragm portion of the chestpiece firmly against the patient's unclothed chest wall. Application of the stethoscope over clothing should be avoided because the breath sounds may be attenuated as they pass through the patient's gown or shirt. Firm pressure is necessary to eliminate chest hair sounds and room noise. Wetting the chest hair can be helpful to minimize extraneous sounds when the hair is thick. Instruct the patient to breathe through an open mouth, deeper and slightly faster than normal. Be sure the patient does not hyperventilate because a reduced carbon dioxide level (hypocapnia) can occur quickly and thus lead to light-headedness and tingling of the lips and fingers. Auscultate anteriorly, laterally, and posteriorly in a systematic manner while comparing side to side (Figure 4-7). Listening posteriorly over the lung bases initially may allow detection of abnormal sounds that may clear with several deep breaths. Compare the sounds heard on one side with sounds heard in the same location on the opposite side. Listen to both inspiration and expiration at each position. Listening to several breaths at any location is necessary when abnormalities are present. Auscultation over the trachea can be particularly helpful in detecting large airway obstruction and in detecting wheezes in some

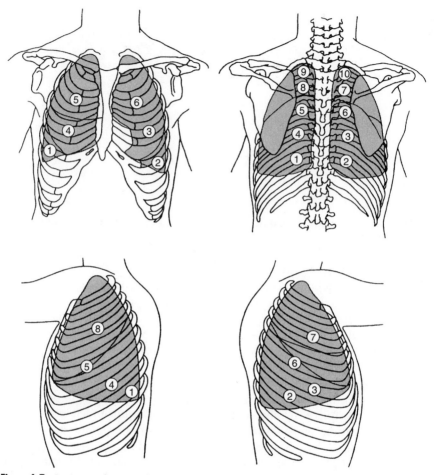

Figure 4-7. Sequence for auscultation of the lungs. *(From Wilkins RL, Dexter JR: Respiratory disease: a case study approach to patient care, ed 2, Philadelphia, 1998, F.A. Davis.)*

patients. Interpretation of lung sounds is described in detail in Chapter 6.

It is also useful to listen to tracheal breath sounds when the peripheral breath sound is reduced or absent. The presence of normal tracheal breath sounds in such cases indicates that the reduced peripheral breath sound is the result of abnormalities in the lung or chest wall.

In critically ill patients, the auscultation findings are potentially very important, yet they can be difficult to obtain. Often the ICU patient is bedridden, unable to cooperate, or even comatose. Furthermore, it is possible that the patient is being mechanically ventilated, which can make it difficult to turn the patient. The examiner should especially make note of the patient's breath sounds in the dependent regions because this is where fluid and mucus initially tend to collect. The examiner may need help in sitting the patient up or turning the patient gently to one side to auscultate the dependent regions.

☞ Key Point

Auscultation of the chest for lung sounds is done by comparing the sounds heard on one side to the sounds heard on the other side at the same location.

Chest Palpation—Lungs

Palpation also can reveal useful information concerning the thorax and lungs. Palpation of the thorax confirms skeletal abnormalities and identifies localized areas of tenderness in the chest wall. Localized tenderness could indicate rib fractures, **costochondritis** (inflammation of the cartilage connecting the ribs to the sternum), and other painful rib lesions. Palpation can reveal masses, pulsations, and areas of **crepitation** (air trapped in the subcutaneous tissue, indicating the presence of subcutaneous emphysema). Subcutaneous air may be present in cases of air leaks caused by severe thoracic injuries and certain procedures (e.g., bronchial rupture and pneumothorax, cardiopulmonary resuscitation, and insertion of chest tubes, lines, and tracheostomy tubes).

The greatest value of palpation, however, may be the sensing of transmitted vibrations through the chest wall. This is also known as **fremitus.** The commonly used forms of fremitus in physical diagnosis are vocal and tactile fremitus. These vibrations are elicited by having the patient say "ninety-nine," "one-two-three," or "eee-eee-eee." Tactile fremitus is perceived by placing the palmar surfaces of your fingers or the palm itself on the chest wall, overlying the lung. Diminished or absent vocal fremitus suggests inability of the lung or chest wall to register or transmit movements of the tracheobronchial air column (e.g., vocal cord failure or airway obstruction). Other conditions that can lead to reduced vibratory or sound transmission include fluid trapped in the pleural space (pleural effusion) and air in the pleural space (pneumothorax).

Tactile fremitus is increased in conditions that tend to increase the density of the lung. Fremitus is better transmitted through a solid, less porous medium such as one would expect in the tissue consolidation of pneumonia. Pleural friction fremitus is the result of pleurisy as the inflamed pleurae rub against each other. The grating sensation of pleural friction fremitus is synchronized with breathing and may be palpable during both phases.

The neck is palpated to identify whether the trachea is in a midline position. The trachea can be deviated to one side as a result of mediastinal tumors, a large unilateral pleural effusion or pneumothorax, or the collapse of an upper lobe. Palpating the thyroid gland and checking for enlarged lymph nodes in the neck (**lymphadenopathy**) is also important.

The peripheral pulses are palpated to detect strength, rhythm, and rate. Weak or absent pulses may indicate poor cardiac function with decreased perfusion. The peripheral pulse may diminish in intensity during inspiration (**paradoxical pulse**) when severe airways obstruction is present (e.g., asthma). This is because of the significant drop in pleural pressure that occurs during inspiration in an effort to cause air to flow through the obstructed airways. The drop in pleural pressure temporarily reduces blood flow out of the thorax, thus causing the peripheral pulse strength to briefly diminish with the corresponding systole.

The abdomen should be palpated to identify whether the liver is enlarged or tender. An enlarged liver is called **hepatomegaly** and is a common finding in patients with right heart failure. A more accurate estimate of the size of the liver can be determined by percussion at the right midclavicular line. The normal vertical span of the liver, in the midclavicular line, varies from 7 cm to 12 cm. In severe emphysema, the lower edge of the liver may be detected by palpation or percussion below the right costal margin because of the downward displacement of the liver from hyperinflation of the lungs. If the total vertical span of the liver is within normal limits, than hepatomegaly is not present. The lower edge of the liver is often difficult to detect by percussion because of the tympanic tone of adjacent bowel. If the lower edge is determined to be below the right costal margin by percussion or palpation, another way to differentiate between downward displacement of the liver and hepatomegaly is to determine the upper border of the liver by percussion: if the upper border is below the sixth intercostal space, in the midclavicular line, downward displacement can be assumed; if it is found at the level of the sixth intercostal space or higher, enlargement is probable. Of course, a pleural effusion around the right lung may lead to dullness to percussion over the inferior portion of the right lung, thus obscuring the border between the lung and the liver.

Chest Percussion—Lungs

Percussion of the chest wall can determine the approximate density of the patient's lungs. The popular method of mediate percussion is learned easily and, if performed properly and systematically, is helpful in certain situations. This method involves placing the distal phalanx of the middle finger of one hand firmly against the chest wall. This finger should be parallel to the ribs in the intercostal spaces. Strike this finger

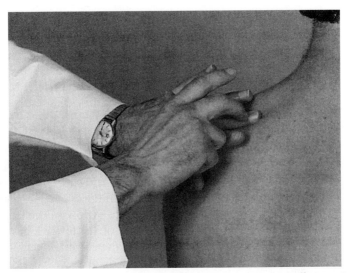

Figure 4-8. Percussion technique: tapping the interphalangeal joint. Only the middle finger of the examiner's nondominant hand should be in contact with the patient's skin surface. *(From Seidel HM, Ball JW, Dains JE, et al: Mosby's guide to physical examination, ed 5, St Louis, 2003, Mosby.)*

with a quick, sharp stroke with the middle finger of the other hand (Figure 4-8). The resulting sounds are classified as normal resonance, increased resonance, or decreased resonance. Normal resonance has a moderately low pitch with a drumlike sound. Increased resonance sounds louder and lower in pitch (e.g., hollow-sounding). The opposite of this, decreased resonance, has a high-pitched, soft sound of shorter duration (e.g., dull- or flat-sounding).

When percussing the lungs, compare similar positions on both sides of the chest. The decreased resonance of pleural fluid, consolidation, or atelectasis is distinct and therefore more obvious than the increased resonance of emphysema or pneumothorax. Unilateral defects are also easier to identify than bilateral abnormalities because there will be a significant difference in the sounds from one side to the other with unilateral disease.

☞ Key Point

Chest percussion for resonance is done to identify major changes in the condition of the underlying lung. Tapping on the chest wall evaluates the resonance of the peripheral portions of the lung and does not reflect the lung condition deeper within the chest.

Inspection and Palpation—Cardiac

The area of the chest wall overlying the heart is known as the **precordium.** It is inspected and palpated for normal and abnormal pulsations. The normal pulsation created by contraction of the left ventricle is called the **point of maximum impulse (PMI)** or **apical impulse.** Normally the PMI is located in the fifth left intercostal space at the midclavicular line. The PMI is often difficult to see or feel in the adult patient because of the buildup of muscle and/or fat or, in female patients, breast tissue.

The PMI tends to shift left or right with abnormalities in the heart or lungs. For example, the PMI shifts leftward with left ventricular hypertrophy and with collapse of the left lower lung. In such cases, the PMI may be felt in the anterior axillary region on the left. Rightward shift of the PMI is seen with collapse of the lower lobes of the right lung. The PMI may be seen or felt in the epigastric region in patients with severe emphysema in which the diaphragm has assumed a low, flat position.

An abnormal pulsation (termed **heave** or **lift**) may be felt at the left sternal border near the fifth intercostal space when the right ventricle is enlarged. This is common in patients who suffer from pulmonary hypertension due to chronic lung disease and is known as *cor pulmonale.* It results from the enlarged right ventricle pounding against the anterior chest wall with each systole. Left ventricular hypertrophy often causes a lift or heave for the same reasons but is located in the anterior or midaxillary region on the left.

Palpation may reveal brief vibrations that coincide with each systole and feel similar to the purring of a cat. These vibrations are produced by the rapid movement of blood through a narrowed pathway and are termed **thrills.** A common cause of a thrill is stenosis of one of the heart valves such as the aortic valve. The thrill associated with aortic stenosis will be felt best over the base or upper portion of the heart during each systole.

☞ Key Point

Right ventricular hypertrophy causes a lift or heave at the left sternal border near the fifth intercostal space. This finding indicates pulmonary hypertension in most cases.

Auscultation—Cardiac

The purpose of cardiac auscultation is to identify the presence and characteristics of normal and abnormal heart sounds. Recognition of abnormal heart sounds requires carefully listening in a quiet room. Prior experience is most helpful when auscultating the heart, especially when the abnormalities are subtle—and they often are. It is helpful to gain an appreciation for normal heart sounds before listening to patients with abnormal findings. Beginning to develop cardiac auscultation skills by listening to the heart sounds of friends first is recommended. This should provide a normal baseline for comparison to later and provide experience in the steps needed for cardiac auscultation.

Complete cardiac auscultation as done in the initial physical examination includes listening to the patient's heart while he or she is sitting, leaning forward, supine, or in the left-lateral decubitus position. Putting the patient in such positions allows the examiner to hear changes in the characteristics of the heart sounds with changes in position. Moving the patient to the left-lateral decubitus position or having him or her lean forward in the sitting position moves the heart closer to the chest wall and should result in louder heart sounds. If such change in position does not result in clearer heart sounds, pleural fluid or other pathology may be present and obscuring the sounds.

Most clinicians performing routine examinations of the patient do not put the patient in all the previously mentioned positions to listen to the heart. Instead, the examination is limited to the sitting and leaning forward or left-lateral decubitus positions, depending on the condition of the patient. Keep in mind that putting the patient in the supine position moves the heart away from the anterior chest wall and may make it difficult to hear faint heart sounds.

☞ Key Point

Having the upright patient lean forward or the supine patient roll on to his or her left side moves the heart closer to the anterior chest wall and should improve the ability to hear the heart sounds.

Once the patient has assumed the proper position for cardiac auscultation, begin the procedure by starting at the apex of the heart and moving upward. At a minimum, listen carefully to the four heart valve regions for at least 15 seconds at each site (Figure 4-9). Do not limit your auscultation to the heart valve areas if you are performing an initial examination or when cardiac abnormalities are strongly suspected. If an abnormality is present at one site, listen to the location longer until the characteristics of the abnormality are noted.

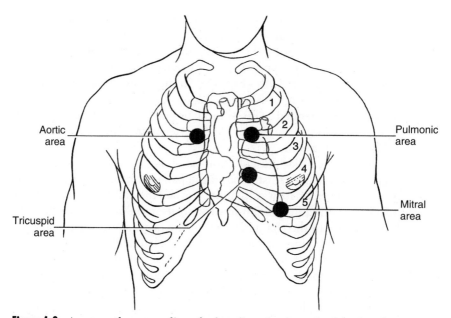

Figure 4-9. Areas on the precordium for best listening to each of the four heart valves. *(From Wilkins RL, Krider SJ, Sheldon RL:* Clinical assessment in respiratory care, *ed 4, St Louis, 2000, Mosby.)*

Repeat the pattern of moving from the apex of the heart to the base of the heart, first with the diaphragm and then with the bell. High-frequency sounds are best heard with the diaphragm, and low-frequency sounds are best heard with the bell (Table 4-5). The normal heart sounds that occur with each cardiac cycle are considered high-frequency sounds. Some abnormal heart sounds, such as the third and fourth heart sounds (see Chapter 7), are considered low-frequency sounds and are best heard with the bell. The adventitious heart sounds (murmurs) can be high or low frequency (see Chapter 7). Murmurs due to stenosis of the aortic valve may radiate to the carotid arteries in the neck.

Table 4-5	Use of the Stethoscope for Cardiac Auscultation
Bell	**Diaphragm**
S3 and S4	S1 and S2
Low-pitched murmurs	High-pitched murmurs

Chapter Highlights

- The medical history is a written account of the events in the patient's life that have relevance to his or her physical and mental health.
- All health care providers must be able to interview the patient to assess the status of his or her symptoms.
- Interviewing is done in the personal space (2 to 4 feet from the patient).
- The initial interview is done to identify the patient's symptoms and past medical history. Subsequent interviews focus on identifying changes in the symptoms that occur in response to treatment.
- Proper eye contact during the interview is an important way to convey interest in the patient.
- A loose productive cough that occurs on a regular basis most of the year suggests chronic bronchitis. Most cases of chronic bronchitis are related to smoking.
- Dyspnea most often occurs in patients with an increase in the work of breathing. Factors that increase the drive to breathe cause dyspnea to increase.
- Chest pain is caused by pleuritic or cardiac disease. Pleuritic pain is increased with breathing and is located laterally. Cardiac pain often is located centrally and is not altered by breathing.
- Rapid and shallow breathing is consistent with a loss of lung volume. The greater the loss of lung volume, the higher the respiratory rate.
- Peripheral cyanosis is consistent with cardiac failure. Central cyanosis indicates respiratory failure.
- Chest auscultation for lung sounds is done by comparing the sounds heard on one side with those heard in the same location on the other side.
- Increased tactile fremitus is caused by lung consolidation. Decreased tactile fremitus is associated with lung hyperinflation and pleural air or fluid.
- Increased resonance with percussion of the chest is heard with lung hyperinflation and with the presence of pleural air (pneumothorax). Decreased resonance is caused by lung consolidation and pleural fluid.
- The normal pulsation seen and felt on the anterior chest is caused by left ventricular contraction. It is called the point of maximum impulse (PMI) or the apical impulse.
- Abnormal pulsations on the anterior chest wall are called heaves or lifts. They often occur with hypertrophy of the left or right ventricle.
- Having the upright patient lean forward or the supine patient roll to the left side will move the heart closer to the anterior chest wall and should result in louder heart sounds.
- Each heart valve is heard best at a specific location on the precordium.

BIBLIOGRAPHY

- Barkauskas VH, Baumann LL, Darling-Fisher CS: *Health and physical assessment*, ed 3, St Louis, 2002, Mosby.
- Seidel HM et al: *Mosby's guide to physical examination*, ed 2, St Louis, 1991, Mosby.

• Wilkins RL, Sheldon RL, Krider SJ: *Clinical assessment in respiratory care,* ed 4, St Louis, 2000, Mosby.

Review Questions

1. In what space is the interview best conducted?
  A. Social space
  B. Personal space
  C. Intimate space
  D. Outer space

2. In what space is conversation with the patient least appropriate?
  A. Social space
  B. Personal space
  C. Intimate space
  D. Outer space

3. Your patient coughs with laughing and exercise. What is a likely cause of the coughing in this case?
  A. Bronchogenic tumor
  B. Asthma
  C. Pleural effusion
  D. Heart failure

4. Sputum production that contains pus is described by what term?
  A. Purulent
  B. Fetid
  C. Copious
  D. None of the above

5. What term is used to describe shortness of breath in the upright position?
  A. Orthopnea
  B. Platypnea
  C. Apnea
  D. Eupnea

6. Which of the following disorders is *not* likely to be associated with hemoptysis?
  A. Mitral stenosis
  B. Pulmonary embolism
  C. Bronchitis
  D. Pericarditis

7. Which of the following characteristics is *not* typical of pleuritic chest pain?
  A. Increases with deep breathing
  B. Radiates to the jaw
  C. Is located laterally
  D. Diminishes with splinting of the affected side

Review Questions—cont'd

8. Which type of pulmonary problem usually causes a breathing pattern with a prolonged expiratory time?

   A. Obstructive lung disease

   B. Atelectasis

   C. Pulmonary edema

   D. Pneumonia

9. Which of the following conditions is least likely to produce jugular venous distention?

   A. Right heart failure

   B. Chronic left heart failure

   C. Chronic hypoxemia

   D. Liver failure

10. True or False

   The diaphragm part of the stethoscope is best for listening to high-pitched sounds.

11. True or False

   It is best to begin chest auscultation of the lung at the apices.

12. Which of the following conditions is associated with increased tactile fremitus?

   A. Pneumonia

   B. Emphysema

   C. Pneumothorax

   D. Pleural effusion

13. Which of the following conditions may result in decreased resonance to percussion?

   A. Pneumothorax

   B. Emphysema

   C. Pneumonia

   D. Asthma

14. What may cause a heave or lift at the left sternal border near the fifth intercostal space?

   A. Pulmonary edema

   B. Pulmonary hypertension

   C. Mitral stenosis

   D. Aortic stenosis

15. How long should you listen to the heart at each of the heart valve areas during a routine physical examination?

   A. 5 seconds

   B. 15 seconds

   C. 30 seconds

   D. 60 seconds

The Stethoscope

After reading this chapter, you will be able to recognize and describe the following:
- Important historical dates and names related to the stethoscope.
- Important features of the modern stethoscope.
- How to clean and care for your stethoscope.

KEY TERMS

binaural	Laennec	Piorry
Bowles	Littmann	stethoscope
Cammann	monaural	

INTRODUCTION

The stethoscope has maintained a position of importance in modern medicine despite the development of more sophisticated diagnostic tools such as radiographs, ultrasonography, and computerized tomography. Although the stethoscope has been around since the early 1800s, it continues to be a popular diagnostic tool because it offers several advantages. It is inexpensive and easy to use, provides immediate feedback, and reveals useful information regarding the patient's diagnosis and response to treatment. The purpose of this chapter is to describe the history of the stethoscope and discuss features of the modern stethoscope.

HISTORY OF THE STETHOSCOPE

Before 1816, auscultation was done by using the direct technique, which called for the physician to place his or her ear directly on the patient's chest. This approach was uncomfortable for both the patient and the doctor, especially if each was of a different gender. In addition, if the patient had poor body hygiene or a contagious disease, the direct technique exposed the doctor to harm.

In 1816, a shy French physician by the name of René Theophile Hyacinthe **Laennec** was presented with an obese female patient with a heart ailment. The circumstances forced Laennec to consider other options for listening to the patient's chest. He remembered from his childhood that sound conducts through cylinders and wondered if rolling up a sheet of paper to create a tube might prove useful. He placed one end of the rolled-up paper against the patient's chest and the other to his ear. To his amazement, he heard the chest sounds better than he had ever heard using the direct technique. From this encounter Laennec rushed off to his workshop, where he developed the first known stethoscope from a block of wood.[1]

Laennec's cylinder of wood was not named at first, but as its popularity grew an official name was needed. After careful thought, he labeled it a **stethoscope** from the Greek words *stethos* and *scope,* meaning "chest" and "examine." His original stethoscope was about 12 inches in length and 2 inches in diameter and was perforated in the middle to allow conduction of sound. It came with a chest piece that was detachable and most useful for heart sounds.[2] The tubular portion of the scope could be divided into two pieces to allow easier storage and transportation (Figure 5-1).

Laennec's stethoscope did not catch on initially but became popular with physicians all over Europe within a few years. Many variations of Laennec's original scope were developed over the ensuing years. Some inventors thought the use of material other than wood, such as metal, or exotic material such as ivory, would be useful. Most initial variations, however, did not improve much on Laennec's original wood cylinder.

☞ Key Point

The first stethoscope was invented by Dr. René Laennec in 1816. This invention improved the value of chest auscultation.

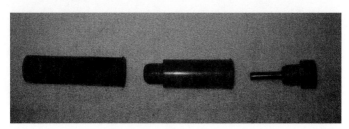

Figure 5-1. Laennec stethoscope from 1819. The end cone was inserted to listen to the heart and removed to listen to the lungs. (*Courtesy of Erik Soiferman, D.O., Medical Antiques Online, www.antiquemed.com.*)

Laennec's original stethoscope and many of the initial variations are known as **monaural** stethoscopes. This name comes from the single-tube design of the instrument. Monaural stethoscopes remained popular for many years because they were easy to use, store, and transport.

An important variation of the monaural stethoscope was developed in 1828 by Pierre Piorry. He developed a trumpet-shaped stethoscope that was made of wood and had removable ivory ear- and chest-pieces. The **Piorry** offered improved interface between the examiner and the scope because of its "custom" earpiece. A similar variation of the Piorry stethoscope is still in use as an obstetrical tool in many countries (Figures 5-2 and 5-3).

A major disadvantage of the monaural stethoscope centered around the fact that only one ear was involved in the auscultation process. This left the other ear to be distracted by noises in the room.

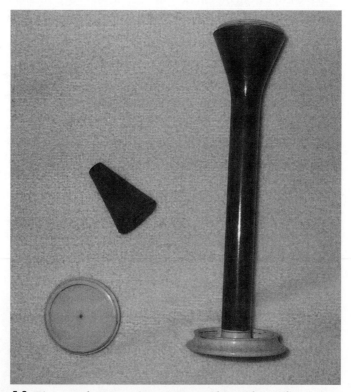

Figure 5-2. Piorry stethoscope, circa 1840, complete with wooden resonator. Piorry was the first to use the "plessimeter" for percussion. His stethoscope was shorter than Laennec's but used the same acoustic principles. *(Courtesy of Erik Soiferman, D.O., Medical Antiques Online, www.antiquemed.com.)*

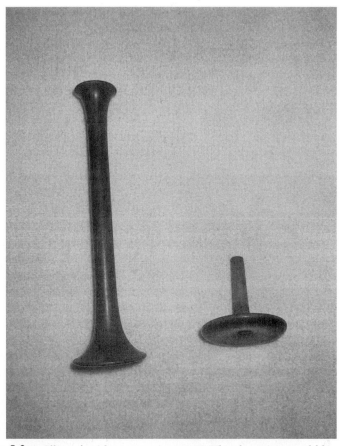

Figure 5-3. Williams' stethoscope, circa 1840. The chestpiece could be stored in either end for ease of use. *(Courtesy of Erik Soiferman, D.O., Medical Antiques Online, www.antiquemed.com.)*

In addition, the interface between the earpiece and the clinician's ear was not optimal for acoustical perception. These problems were overcome by the development of a stethoscope that employed both ears with properly fitting earpieces. These types of scopes are called **binaural** stethoscopes and they came on the medical scene in the 1850s. They offer the advantage of minimizing the interference of room noise during auscultation. In addition, the earpieces of binaural stethoscopes provided an improved fit, which enhanced the ability to detect heart and lung sounds.

The first commercially successful binaural stethoscope is credited to Dr. George **Cammann** of New York in 1855. Dr. Cammann did not have the initial idea for such a stethoscope but did produce the first one that became popular. Cammann's model had ivory earpieces connected to metal tubes. The tubes were covered by wound silk and attached to a hollow ball intended to amplify sounds. The ball was attached to a conical, bell chestpiece (Figure 5-4). Cammann's binaural stethoscope had the basic design that is still popular today. Today, however, rubber tubing has replaced the metal tubes, providing better flexibility of the stethoscope while maintaining excellent acoustical conductance.

☞ Key Point

The first binaural stethoscope became commercially available in 1855. It was developed by Dr. George Cammann.

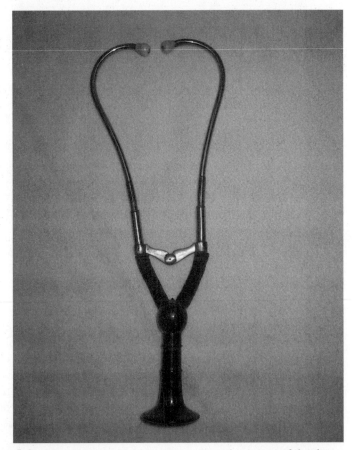

Figure 5-4. Cammann stethoscope, circa 1855. This is one of the three oldest examples. *(Courtesy of Erik Soiferman, D.O., Medical Antiques Online, www.antiquemed.com.)*

The next major development in the progress of stethoscopes came at about 1910. All stethoscopes before this date used a bell chestpiece for interfacing between the patient and the stethoscope. The bell was great for listening to low-pitched sounds but inadequate for some heart sounds and many lung sounds, which are higher pitched. This problem was overcome with the development of the diaphragm chestpiece. The first diaphragm chestpiece employed a membrane stretched over the bell and was designed to allow better auscultation of higher-pitched sounds. The first popular stethoscope to employ the use of a diaphragm in the chestpiece was the **Bowles** model (Figure 5-5). Later, in 1926, Howard Sprague designed the first stethoscope that employed

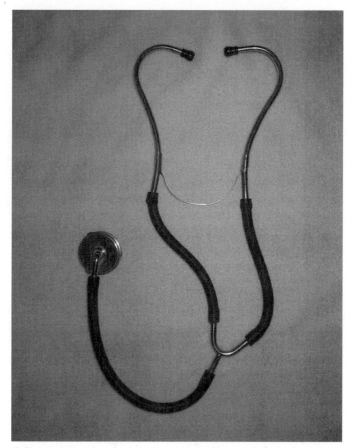

Figure 5-5. Bowles stethoscope, circa 1900. Bowles model was the first popular model to use a diaphragm chestpiece. *(Courtesy of Erik Soiferman, D.O., Medical Antiques Online, www.antiquemed.com.)*

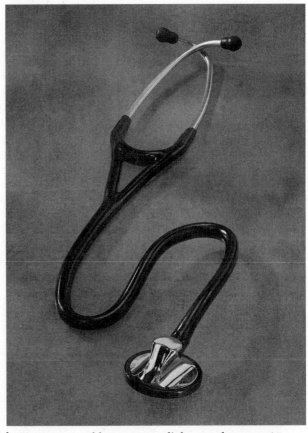

Figure 5-6. Littmann tunable, master cardiology stethoscope. *(Courtesy of 3M.)*

a chestpiece with separate bell and diaphragm. Today this design is very popular; however, **Littmann** 3M has produced a tunable stethoscope with a single chestpiece that can serve as a bell or diaphragm depending on how much pressure is applied. Light pressure will result in the chestpiece functioning as a bell and firm pressure causes it to serve as a diaphragm (Figure 5-6).

Littmann also has developed an electronic stethoscope that is capable of many functions. It can record a patient's heart or lung sounds and allows the recording to be downloaded to a desktop computer for analysis and storage. Storing the patient's lung or heart sounds allows for analysis of the sounds over time. The scope also can determine and display the patient's heart rate (Figure 5-7).

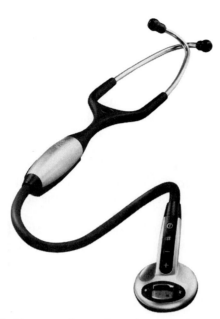

Figure 5-7. Littmann electronic stethoscope. *(Courtesy of 3M.)*

☞ Key Point

The first stethoscope to employ a diaphram was produced in 1910 and was known as the *Bowles model*. It was designed to improve auscultation of higher-pitched sounds, such as lung sounds and many heart sounds.

FEATURES OF A MODERN STETHOSCOPE

Numerous features should be considered in choosing a stethoscope:
1. Length of the tubing
2. Comfort of the earpieces
3. Chestpiece design and functions
4. Single versus double tubing

The stethoscope should have tubing that is 18 to 26 inches in length. Shorter tubing may be better at transmitting sound but is inconvenient in reaching the patient's chest. Longer tubing may reduce sound transmission due to increased attenuation.

The earpieces should be made of a material that easily conforms to the clinician's ear canals. Hard plastic is uncomfortable, and very soft rubber breaks down over time. A softer plastic material is most useful. The metal tubes that connect the earpieces to the rubber tubing should be adjustable so that the clinician can angle the earpieces forward to better conform to his or her outer ear canal for comfort and improved ability to hear chest sounds.

The chestpiece should have both a bell and diaphragm or have a tunable chestpiece that allows auscultation of both high and low-pitched sounds. The bell is useful for listening for an S3 and/or S4 and the low-pitched diastolic rumble of mitral insufficiency, and the diaphragm is useful for lung sounds, S1, S2, and most heart murmurs. Clinicians who care for pediatric and older patients should purchase a stethoscope that offers multiple chestpieces of different sizes—one small enough for the very young and larger chestpieces for adults. The mechanism for switching from use of the bell to the diaphragm should be easy to operate.

Whether single or double tubing is better for acoustical transmission of sound is unclear. The stethoscope with double tubing may offer better sound transmission at very little extra cost.

CLEANING AND MAINTAINING THE STETHOSCOPE

The stethoscope can harbor pathogens and could serve as a source of infections when applied to different patients without proper cleaning after each encounter.[3–5] The use of isopropyl alcohol swabs or ethyl alcohol gel to wipe down the chest piece and under the rim of the diaphragm between patient encounters is recommended for clinicians working within the hospital setting.[3] Frequent cleaning of the stethoscope is especially needed when clinicians care for patients with surgical wounds, chest tubes, or catheters that put the patient at higher risk of nosocomial infection. The use of warm soapy water is not effective for killing many of the pathogens that are found in the hospital setting.[3,5] In the outpatient setting, where low-risk patients are seen, less frequent cleaning of the stethoscope seems reasonable.

The earpieces should be cleaned regularly to prevent the build-up of ear wax and dirt that may interfere with auscultation. The application of warm soapy water should be adequate for such purposes. The diaphragm portion of the chestpiece and tubing should be checked periodically for cracks or other defects that may hinder function.

☞ Key Point

The stethoscope can pass bacteria from one patient to the next if it is not cleaned effectively between patient encounters. The use of 70% isopropyl alcohol or ethyl alcohol gel appears to be effective as a cleaning agent because it destroys most of the bacteria encountered.

Chapter Highlights

- The first stethoscope was invented by Dr. René Laennec in 1816. The first stethoscope was made from a block of hollowed-out wood.
- Single-tube stethoscopes are called monaural stethoscopes.
- The Piorry stethoscope was developed in 1828 and offered removable ear- and chest-pieces.
- Binaural stethoscopes came on the scene in the 1850s and allowed examiners to use both ears when listening to the heart or lungs.
- The first commercially successful binaural stethoscope is credited to Dr. George Cammann of New York in 1855.
- The first stethoscope to employ a diaphragm chestpiece was introduced around 1910. This allowed better auscultation of higher-pitched sounds.
- The ideal modern stethoscope should be about 18 to 24 inches in length, have comfortable earpieces, include a bell and diaphragm (or a tunable chestpiece), and be an excellent conductor of sound.
- Stethoscopes used to assess critically ill patients at high risk for infection should be cleaned with isopropyl alcohol or ethyl alcohol gel after each patient encounter.

REFERENCES

1. Abdulla R: History of the stethoscope, *Ped Cardiol* 22:371-372, 2001.
2. Jay V: The legacy of Laennec, *Arch Pathol Lab Med* 124:1420-1421, 2000.
3. Marinella MA, Pierson C, Chenoweth C: The stethoscope: a potential source of nosocomial infection? *Arch Intern Med* 157:786-790, 1997.
4. Jones JS, Hoerle D: Stethoscopes: a potential vector of infection? *Annals Emerg Med* 26:296-299, 1995.
5. Nunez S, Moreno A, Green K, Villar J: The stethoscope in the emergency department: a vector of infection? *Epidemiol Infect* 124:233-237, 2000.

Review Questions

1. Who is credited with inventing the first stethoscope?
   A. Laennec
   B. Cammann
   C. Marsh
   D. Piorry

2. What material was used to create the first stethoscope?
   A. Metal
   B. Plastic
   C. Ivory
   D. Wood

Continued

Review Questions—cont'd

3. Who is credited with developing the first monaural stethoscope with custom earpieces?
   A. Laennec
   B. Cammann
   C. Piorry
   D. Bowles

4. Who is credited with developing the first commercially available binaural stethoscope?
   A. Laennec
   B. Cammann
   C. Piorry
   D. Bowles

5. What model of stethoscope was the first to use a diaphragm chestpiece?
   A. Bowles model
   B. Marsh model
   C. Cammann model
   D. Piorry model

6. What company has developed a tunable chestpiece that serves as a diaphragm and bell depending on how much pressure is applied?
   A. General Electric
   B. Littmann 3M
   C. Sprague Company
   D. Biosystems

7. What is the ideal length of tubing for the stethoscope?
   A. 12 to 16 inches
   B. 16 to 20 inches
   C. 18 to 26 inches
   D. 24 to 36 inches

8. True or False
   Isopropyl alcohol swabs have been shown to be effective in eliminating most pathogens from the modern stethoscope.

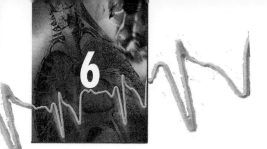

Lung Sounds

6

OBJECTIVES

After reading this chapter, you will be able to recognize and describe the following:

- The appropriate terms for describing normal and abnormal lung sounds.
- The proposed mechanisms thought to be responsible for production of normal and abnormal lung sounds.
- The significance of normal breath sound intensity at any chest wall location and potential causes for reduction in intensity.
- The relationship between breath sound intensity and the degree of chronic obstructive lung disease.
- The therapy that may be indicated by decreased breath sounds, bronchial breath sounds, late-inspiratory or coarse crackles, wheezes, and stridor.
- The characteristics of crackles and wheezes that should be evaluated and how these characteristics change with lung disease.
- The mechanisms for bronchophony, egophony, and whispered pectoriloquy.

KEY TERMS

adventitious lung sounds	crackles	tracheobronchial breath sounds
bone crepitus	egophony	vesicular breath sounds
bronchial breath sounds	pleural friction rub	wheeze
bronchophony	rales	whispered pectoriloquy
bronchovesicular breath sounds	rhonchi	xiphi-sternal crunch
	stridor	
	tracheal breath sounds	

L ung sounds can be divided into two major categories: breath sounds and adventitious lung sounds. Breath sounds are normal noises that can be heard on the chest wall with breathing. **Adventitious lung sounds** are abnormal sounds superimposed on the breath sounds and usually indicate some type of respiratory disorder. First, this chapter will focus on the terminology, mechanisms, and interpretation of normal and abnormal breath sounds; a similar review for the adventitious lung sounds will follow.

BREATH SOUNDS

Terminology for Breath Sounds

Normal breath sounds have traditionally been divided into four types: tracheal, bronchial, bronchovesicular, and vesicular (see Figure 6-1 for a diagrammatic representation of these sounds). Directly over the trachea, the breath sound is particularly loud and high pitched; it is described as **tracheal.** The tracheal breath sound has a pause between the inspiratory and expiratory components, and the expiratory component is slightly longer. The term **bronchial** is used to describe a similar sound that is also harsh and high pitched with approximately equal inspiratory and expiratory components. This sound may be heard directly over a major bronchus during normal breathing. Because tracheal and bronchial breath sounds are very similar in characteristics, we prefer to use the term **tracheobronchial** to refer to these loud, tubular-type breath sounds. **Bronchovesicular** sounds are a slight variation to the tracheobronchial sound and are heard just distal to the central airways. They are less intense (softer) and lower pitched than bronchial sounds but maintain an equal

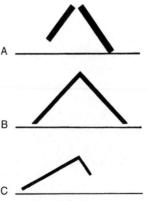

Figure 6-1. Diagrams of normal breath sounds. **A,** Tracheal; **B,** bronchovesicular; **C,** vesicular. The upstroke represents inspiration, and the down stroke represents expiration. The thickness of the line represents the intensity of the sound and the angle between the upstroke, and the horizontal line represents pitch. The length of the line represents duration.

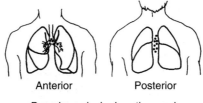

Bronchovesicular breath sounds

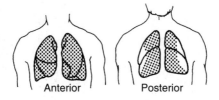

Vesicular breath sounds

Figure 6-2. Location on the chest wall where normal vesicular breath sounds are heard.

inspiratory and expiratory component (see Figure 6-1). The **vesicular breath sound** is significantly softer in intensity and is primarily an inspiratory sound. The expiratory component of the vesicular breath sound is normally minimal, only occurring during the initial one-third of the expiratory phase. The vesicular breath sound is normally heard over all areas of the chest distal to the central airways (Figure 6-2).

The term *vesicular* is derived from the Latin word for small vessels. Use of the term originated when clinicians thought this sound resulted from air entry into the small vessels (alveoli). We now know, however, that the peripheral lung units in healthy individuals are essentially silent.

When vesicular breath sounds are found to be of less intensity than expected, they are described as *diminished* (reduced) or even absent in extreme cases. If the peripheral breath sound increases in intensity, it is described as *harsh;* if it also takes on a more prominent expiratory component, it is described as tracheobronchial (tubular) or bronchial.

☞ Key Point

The normal vesicular breath sound is a soft, low-pitched sound heard primarily during inspiration.

Mechanisms of Breath Sounds

The exact mechanism(s) responsible for production of normal breath sounds is unknown. The normal breath sounds are believed to be produced primarily by turbulent flow in the larger airways; however, the inspiratory phase of the vesicular breath sound is believed to be produced more distally than the expiratory phase. Because more peripheral airways normally maintain laminar flow, they are not believed to be responsible for significant sound production. They may play a role in the transmission of the turbulent sounds of the larger airways to the peripheral chest. The majority of experimental evidence suggests that normal breath sounds are produced regionally within each lung and probably within each lobe.[1] This implies, for example, that the breath sounds heard over a specific lobe are probably a result of air entry into that underlying lobe.

As described in Chapters 1 and 3, the normal breath sound is attenuated as it passes through healthy lung tissue. It alters the tracheobronchial sounds of the central airways to a softer version with a lower pitch. Changes in lung pathology will alter the sound transmission characteristics of the lung parenchyma. Diseases that increase lung density will usually increase the sound transmission qualities and result in a significant decrease in the filtering effect. As a result, tracheobronchial (tubular) breath sounds may be heard over areas of consolidation (as with lobar pneumonia or atelectasis), provided a patent bronchus is present (Figure 6-3). An obstructed bronchus (by a mucus plug, for example) will block transmission of the bronchial sounds and lead to absent or markedly diminished breath sounds over the affected region.

Diminished breath sounds may result from decreases in sound generation (less turbulent flow) with shallow breathing patterns. This may occur with neuromuscular diseases and other restrictive lung defects. Obstructive lung disease may also result in diminished breath sounds when airflow limitation is severe. Diminished breath sounds will also be identified when the sound transmission ability of the lung or chest wall is reduced and results in more attenuation of the turbulent flow sounds. This can occur when the lung becomes hyperinflated (as with emphysema), with pleural disease (effusion or pneumothorax), or with muscular and obese chest walls (see Figure 6-3). Finally, sound transmission through the lung will be reduced when mucus plugging of the airways is present.

☞ Key Point

The primary source of all normal breath sounds is the turbulent flow that occurs in the larger airways.

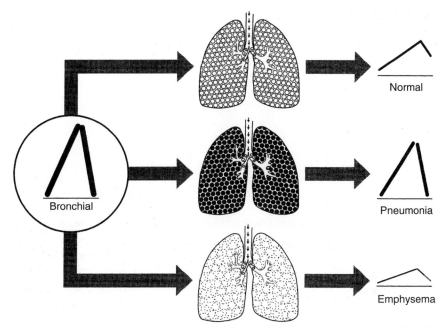

Figure 6-3. Influence of various changes in lung density on the perception of breath sounds. Normal lung *(top)* reduces the bronchial breath sound to a normal vesicular breath sound that is softer and lower pitched. Lung consolidation *(middle)* causes little attenuation of the bronchial breath sound. Lung hyperinflation *(bottom)* causes significant attenuation of the bronchial breath sound and results in diminished breath sounds. *(From Wilkins RL, Krider SJ, Sheldon RL: Clinical assessment in respiratory care, ed 4, St Louis, 2000, Mosby.)*

Interpretation of Breath Sounds

An important aspect of auscultation is the process of identifying the intensity of the vesicular breath sound. This requires that clinicians have an appreciation for the expected normal breath sound intensity (BSI). Through experience, the ability to recognize significant abnormalities in BSI becomes easier. Comparing one side to another is helpful in recognizing unilateral defects. Slight variation from one side to the other, however, is within normal limits.[2]

Normal BSI at a single location on the chest wall correlates with the degree of ventilation in the underlying lobe. A normal BSI in the adult implies that underlying regional ventilation is occurring, but the exact degree cannot be determined. A decrease in BSI may be the result of diminished ventilation in the underlying lobe, poor sound transmission qualities of the lung, or both of these factors. Diminished regional ventilation may occur with bronchial intubation, mucus plugging, or bronchial obstruction. Poor sound transmission qualities of the lung occur with hyperinflation, as in acute or chronic airway obstruction.

☞ Key Point

Normal breath sounds at any location on the chest wall implies that ventilation of the underlying lobe is present.

In cases of airway obstruction, decreased ventilation and sound transmission contribute to diminished BSI. Therapy such as postural drainage, bronchial hygiene techniques, and bronchodilators may result in better regional ventilation and BSI in affected areas. Therapy that results in a reversal of airway obstruction and diminished hyperinflation should result in a more normal BSI. This improvement is more likely to occur in asthma and bronchitis than in emphysema because the changes that cause airway obstruction in asthma (e.g., bronchospasm) and bronchitis (e.g., thick mucus) are more reversible.

Evaluating the BSI over multiple sites on the chest wall can help determine the degree of chronic airflow obstruction. Studies have shown a good correlation between BSI scores and expiratory flow parameters from spirograms.[3–5] This requires estimating the BSI on a scale of 0 to 3 in which 0 = absent, 1 = diminished, 2 = normal, and 3 = louder than normally expected. This examination is made at six locations on the chest wall: bilaterally over the upper anterior regions, in the midaxillae, and at the posterior bases. BSI scores are then tabulated and correlated with pulmonary function results.

Results have shown that normal BSI scores nearly always rule out the presence of severe airway obstruction. Definitely reduced BSI scores are strong indications of severe airway obstruction. Mild to moderate obstructive defects are not quantified easily with this method because patients with moderate reduction in BSI scores have a variety of pulmonary function results.

These results suggest that when the history or physical examination implies chronic airway obstruction, careful evaluation of the breath sounds may help quantify the degree of obstruction present. Preoperative patients with moderate to severe reductions in BSI scores should have spirograms to evaluate further the pulmonary system and its ability to tolerate the planned surgery.

☞ **Key Point**

Reduced breath sounds are the result of either reduced sound production (as occurs with shallow breathing) or reduced sound transmission through the lung or chest wall or both.

The amount of variability in the breath sounds of healthy subjects has been found to be insignificant from one breath to the next.[6] In addition, Mahagnah found that the variance in breath sounds over a 7-day period was not significant in healthy people.[7] Clinicians can expect that the breath sounds of their patients should not significantly change from one breath to the next and from one day to the next unless pathological alterations in the lung are occurring. Changes in the breath sounds at the same location over the peripheral lung from one day to the next are not normal and probably represent changes in lung pathology.

Evaluating the expiratory component of the vesicular breath sound is important. Normally, it is faint and heard only during the early part of exhalation. For this reason, it is often ignored. One of the first signs of lung congestion is a change in the vesicular breath sound to more of a tracheobronchial sound. In such cases, the breath sound increases in pitch and intensity and the expiratory component of the breath sound becomes more prominent. This change is subtle and often missed. It occurs initially in the dependent regions of the lungs in the bedridden patient. Because these areas on the chest wall are difficult to assess, especially in the comatose patient, this abnormality often is not detected until more obvious abnormalities are present.

Lung expansion therapies and/or postural drainage may be indicated when tracheobronchial-type breath sounds are detected over the lung fields. The breath sound should return to a more vesicular type if the therapy results in reexpansion of the atelectatic regions.

Although the chest roentgenogram has become the cornerstone of chest assessment, its diagnostic yield is low in many cases. Evaluating the breath sounds may, in some cases, allow omission of a routine chest roentgenogram. Normal breath sounds in patients with respiratory complaints or fever ruled out pneumonia with greater than 95% certainty in one study.[8] This suggests that careful attention to the patient's breath sounds may allow for a reduction in unnecessary radiation exposure and costs.

☞ **Key Point**

Bronchial breath sounds heard over the lung suggest that the sound attenuation properties of the normal lung have been altered because of an increase in lung density.

ADVENTITIOUS LUNG SOUNDS

Terminology for Adventitious Lung Sounds

Based on acoustical recordings and analysis of lung sounds, the adventitious lung sounds (ALS) can be divided into two categories: continuous and discontinuous. Continuous ALS are musical sounds with a constant pitch. Their duration may range from a very short time (200 msec) to several seconds. They are more often heard during exhalation and are associated with obstruction of airways. Discontinuous ALS are intermittent, crackling or bubbling sounds of short duration (<20 msec). These brief bursts of sound are heard most commonly during inspiration and may be present with both restrictive and obstructive defects.

The terms used to describe ALS lack standardization even today.[9] Originally Laennec used the term **rales** for all abnormal sounds, distinguishing four subgroups: moist, mucous, sonorous, and sibilant. When patients associated *rale* with *death rattle,* Laennec recommended use of the more neutral term *rhonchus* (the Greek synonym). Later his work was translated into English, and the words *rales* and ***rhonchi*** were used differently, thus increasing confusion. Even today, much disagreement remains with regard to the correct terms to be used in describing commonly heard sounds.[9]

A major part of the terminology confusion centers around use of the terms *rales* and *rhonchi*.[10] Rather than give new definitions to these old terms, we will follow the recommendation of others[11–12] and suggest that discontinuous ALS be described as **crackles** and continuous ALS as **wheezes** (Table 6-1). The high-pitched, continuous sound heard over the upper airway of a patient with upper airway obstruction is called **stridor**. The clinical significance for each of these sounds will be discussed in the following pages.

☞ Key Point

Adventitious lung sounds can be divided into continuous and discontinuous. The discontinuous type are best described with the term *crackles* and the continuous type with the term *wheeze*.

Qualifying Adjectives

The terms used to qualify the adventitious lung sounds also lack standardization. This may explain why few clinicians use adjectives to describe lung sounds.[9,13] Experts now suggest using adjectives that have a scientific basis consistent with waveform analysis of the acoustical

Table 6-1	Terminology for Adventitious Lung Sounds (ALS)	
Classification	Suggested Term	Terms Used Previously
Discontinuous	Crackles	Rales, crepitations
High pitched	Fine crackles	Dry rales
Low pitched	Coarse crackles	Wet rales
Continuous	Wheeze	Musical rales
High pitched	Wheeze	Sibilant rales
Low pitched	Low-pitched wheeze	Rhonchi, sonorous rales

characteristics. Terms such as *wet, dry, sonorous,* and *sibilant,* which have no acoustical basis, should be replaced with more accurate terms such as *high pitched, low pitched, fine, medium,* and *coarse.* We will use the terms *fine, medium,* and *coarse* to indicate the pitch of discontinuous abnormal lung sounds. For example, *fine crackles* would imply high-pitched sounds and *coarse crackles* would imply *low-pitched sounds.* We will use *mild, moderate,* and *severe* to indicate the intensity of continuous abnormal lung sounds, such as wheezes. The terms *high pitched* and *low pitched* will be used also to describe continuous ALS.

A more important description of diagnostic value is the timing of the ALS during the respiratory cycle.[14] Abnormal sounds should be described as *inspiratory, expiratory,* or both. In addition, the specific timing during inspiration (e.g., late-inspiratory crackles) may be of some help. The clinical significance of such descriptions is explained more extensively in the following discussion.

☞ Key Point

The qualifying adjectives used to describe ALS should have an acoustical basis. Terms such as *high pitched* and *low pitched* are acceptable. Terms such as *wet* or *dry* have no acoustical basis and are not acceptable.

Mechanisms of Adventitious Lung Sounds

Discontinuous ALS are probably produced by more than one mechanism. Two commonly accepted theories suggest that crackles can be produced by the bubbling of air through airway secretions or by the sudden opening of small airways. Crackles associated with the movement of airway secretions in larger airways are typically coarse and may occur during both inspiration and expiration. They may clear with suctioning or effective coughing.

Crackles associated with the sudden opening of airways may be produced by a rapid equalization of pressure between patent and collapsed airways. These crackles are inspiratory sounds, which may occur when peripheral airways pop open as collapsed (atelectatic) regions are inflated (Figure 6-4). With atelectasis due to a shallow breathing pattern, the crackles often disappear after a few deep breaths or after changes in position; whereas with pulmonary fibrosis, the crackles persist. In mild pulmonary fibrosis, the crackles are predominantly heard late in inspiration but may become paninspiratory with an end-inspiratory accentuation as the disease progresses. Late-inspiratory crackles are often repetitive with several respiratory cycles and initially identified in dependent lung zones. Late-inspiratory crackles strongly suggest a restrictive lung defect and indicate a loss in lung volume.

More proximal airways may collapse during exhalation when bronchial wall compliance increases. During the subsequent inspiration, the airways will pop open intermittently and produce unique inspiratory crackles. In such cases, the crackles primarily occur early in inspiration and may not be affected by coughing or changes in position. Early-inspiratory crackles are scanty, low pitched, and audible at the mouth as well as over the chest. They could suggest chronic obstructive airway diseases that affect bronchial wall compliance.

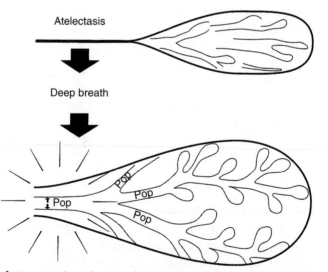

Figure 6-4. Proposed mechanism for late-inspiratory crackles. Peripheral airways pop open when inspiratory effort is sufficient to overcome the forces causing atelectasis. *(From Wilkins RL, Krider SJ, Sheldon RL:* Clinical assessment in respiratory care, *ed 4, St Louis, 2000, Mosby.)*

☞ Key Point

Crackles are believed to be produced by the sudden opening of collapsed airways and with the movement of excessive airway secretions.

Continuous ALS are believed to result from airway narrowing, which initially causes rapid airflow through the site of obstruction. The more rapid airflow decreases lateral airway wall pressures and results in the opposite walls pulling closer together and briefly touching. As a result, flow is briefly interrupted, and airway pressure increases. The airway now returns to a more open position, permitting airflow to return (Figure 6-5). The cycle repeats itself rapidly, causing vibration of airway walls. This process will continue until insufficient flow occurs, as when the patient tires, or until the airway obstruction is relieved.

The pitch of the continuous adventitious sound is determined by the relationship between flow and degree of obstruction. More rapid flows or tighter obstruction result in higher-pitched sounds. Lower flows or less obstruction will result in lower-pitched sounds.

The timing of the continuous ALS can provide important clues as to the location of the airway abnormality. During expiration, intrathoracic airways become progressively narrower. This is accentuated when intrathoracic pressures increase during forced breathing, as when the patient actively forces the air out of the chest. As a result, the process of producing continuous adventitious lung sounds is likely to occur more frequently and for longer periods during expiration, when variable intrathoracic obstruction is present. The opposite is true during inspiration, when negative intrapleural pressures cause intrathoracic airways to widen.

A variable obstruction of extrathoracic airways (e.g., trachea, larynx) will result more often in continuous adventitious lung sounds during inspiration. This occurs because airway pressure distal to the obstruction is decreased significantly in relation to atmospheric pressure outside the airway during inspiration. This pressure gradient narrows the site of obstruction further and sets up the situation needed to produce inspiratory stridor or wheeze. During expiration, a rising airway pressure produces a pressure gradient that is positive from inside to outside of the airway, and the extrathoracic obstruction lessens. Thus extrathoracic airway obstruction is less likely to result in continuous adventitious lung sounds during expiration. If the obstruction becomes fixed or severe enough, stridor will be heard during inspiration and expiration, regardless of the location of the obstruction.

It is important to note that only the larger bronchi are capable of generating continuous adventitious lung sounds. Small airways have

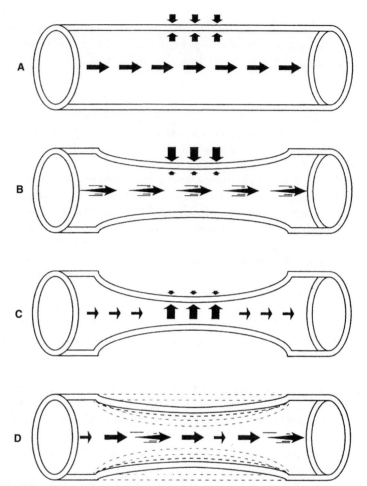

Figure 6-5. Proposed mechanism for wheezes. **A,** Normal airway, where internal and external airway wall pressures are equal; **B,** slight narrowing of the airway, which causes an increase in the velocity of airflow and a decrease in the lateral wall pressure inside the airway relative to outside; **C,** greater narrowing of the airway to the point that forward airflow is inhibited and lateral wall pressure increases relative to outside pressure; and **D,** fluttering of the airway walls between position **B** and **C.** *(From Wilkins RL, Krider SJ, Sheldon RL: Clinical assessment in respiratory care, ed 4, St Louis, 2000, Mosby.)*

significantly lower flows than the larger airways and are much less likely to be a source of expiratory wheezes. Only two or three peripheral generations of bronchial airways past the segmental bronchi are believed to be capable of producing continuous sounds.

Key Point

Narrowing of intrathoracic airways is more likely to result in expiratory wheezing.

Pleural Friction Rub

Normally, the smooth, moist layers of the pleura slide silently on one another during breathing. Alterations in the pleura from inflammation or fibrin deposits can result in added friction between the pleural layers. The sound produced is usually nonmusical and has been compared to the creaking sound of old leather or to the sound produced by rubbing two inflated balloons together. This sound is called a **pleural friction rub.** Friction rubs are usually lower-pitched, are of longer duration than pulmonary crackles and are commonly present during both inspiration and expiration; however, they may be mistaken for sounds emanating from within the lung. Technically, rubs are not lung sounds.

Interpretation of Adventitious Lung Sounds

Crackles

An important aspect to consider when evaluating crackles is their timing during the respiratory cycle. Diffuse paninspiratory or late-inspiratory crackles highly suggest a restrictive lung defect. This may occur with asbestosis, atelectasis, pulmonary fibrosis, congestive heart failure (CHF), or pneumonia. Crackles are rare in sarcoidosis.[15] Late-inspiratory crackles are usually superimposed on a harsh or bronchial breath sound. With atelectasis, the crackles tend to be gravity dependent and commonly clear with several deep breaths, changes in position, or coughing.

Patients with interstitial pneumonia or fibrosis typically have fine late-inspiratory crackles.[14,16] They appear to be related to the severity of the illness. In early stages, the crackles may be heard only in the bases; however, they progress to the upper lobes with advancing disease.

Late-inspiratory crackles may be reversible in certain clinical conditions, such as atelectasis, pneumonia, and CHF. Therapy that reexpands atelectatic regions, such as continuous positive airway pressure (CPAP), incentive spirometry, and repositioning of the patient should help resolve the crackles in these situations. In CHF patients, diuretics also may help. With pulmonary fibrosis, the inspiratory crackles persist in spite of deep breaths because they are a result of permanent pathologic changes in the lung.

☞ **Key Point**

Fine, late-inspiratory crackles strongly suggest restrictive lung disease.

Early-inspiratory crackles may be identified in patients with chronic obstructive pulmonary disease (COPD). In such cases, the crackles are scanty and often radiate to the mouth. They are generally not affected by coughing or changes in position. Their presence may indicate severe obstructive disease. Patients with COPD may have crackles during any part of inspiration; they are usually found in only a few locations over the chest[16] and may indicate more severe disease.

Early-inspiratory crackles are not likely to be affected by therapy because the mechanisms responsible for them (altered bronchial wall compliance and elastic recoil) are the result of more permanent alterations in lung pathology.

Coarse, gurgling crackles indicate excessive airway secretions. In this situation, the crackles tend to occur in both inhalation and exhalation as air moves across the secretions. Gurgling crackles usually will clear with an effective cough or with tracheal suctioning. They are most often present in patients with a diminished cough caused by artificial airways, neuromuscular diseases, or medications.

Coarse inspiratory crackles are a common finding in bronchiectasis. The crackles of bronchiectasis typically are located early- to mid-inspiration and are more profuse than in chronic bronchitis and emphysema.[17] They tend to become less in number after coughing.

☞ **Key Point**

Coarse inspiratory and expiratory crackles occur when excessive airway secretions are present. They may clear with coughing.

Inspiratory crackles are generally considered an abnormality but may be identified in patients with normal lungs in certain situations. Profuse inspiratory crackles have been identified in healthy subjects during inhalation following a maximal exhalation.[18] They are rarely identified during breathing from the resting lung volume in healthy individuals. Therefore inspiratory crackles should be considered an abnormality only when they occur during inspiration from a resting lung volume.

Crackles may be difficult to hear in patients who are obese, especially when the crackles are not loud. They may also be underappreciated when the vesicular breath sound is louder, as occurs with deep and fast breathing.[19] For this reason, having the patient breathe slowly and deeply may offer an advantage when inspiratory crackles are suspected.

Wheezes

Several characteristics of the wheeze should be identified when present. Wheezes may be classified as high pitched or low pitched, inspiratory or expiratory, short or long, and single or multiple. Identifying these characteristics will help determine the severity and location of the airway obstruction and the response to therapy. Changes in these characteristics may be subtle and go unnoticed if auscultation is done too rapidly.

The pitch of the wheeze is a function of the relationship between the degree of airway obstruction and the flow of air past the obstruction. In the patient with good respiratory effort, the pitch of the wheeze increases as the airway obstruction worsens. If the patient tires and respiratory effort is diminished, tighter airway obstruction may result in lower inspiratory and expiratory flows and lower-pitched wheezes (or none at all). The intensity of the sound will also be decreased in such cases.

Braughman and Loudon[20] have documented that improvements in expiratory flows (FEV_1) in asthmatics treated with bronchodilators are associated with a reduction in the sound frequency of the wheeze. Hence, bronchodilator therapy may lower the pitch of the wheeze if treatment is effective. Other clinical parameters, such as the vital signs, will help confirm that the reduction in pitch is the result of bronchodilation and not respiratory failure.

The timing of the wheeze during the respiratory cycle may provide clues as to the location and severity of obstruction. As mentioned previously, inspiratory stridor more commonly is associated with extrathoracic lesions, such as laryngeal narrowing from a tumor or postextubation inflammation, and expiratory wheezing more commonly is associated with intrathoracic lesions, such as asthma.[21] Exceptions do occur. A bronchial tumor or foreign body aspiration that produces a fixed airway obstruction typically results in both inspiratory and expiratory wheezing. It is not uncommon for patients with chronic bronchitis, bronchiectasis, or cystic fibrosis to have both inspiratory and expiratory wheezes. Inspiratory wheezes may be heard after a series of crackles in fibrosing lung diseases. The wheezing in this situation usually occurs late in inspiration.

Studies have documented a relationship between the proportion of the respiratory cycle occupied by wheezing and flow parameters.[20,22] Asthmatic patients in these studies were treated with bronchodilators; as expiratory flow parameters improved, the proportion of the respiratory cycle in which wheezing occurred was reduced. For example, wheezing may be heard during both inspiration and expiration or be pan-expiratory before treatment. After treatment, if obstruction is improved, the wheezing may be heard only during the last half of expiration, occupying a shorter portion of the respiratory cycle. Precise evaluation of changes in wheezing duration is not possible without phonopneumography, but extremes are recognized easily with auscultation.

✍ Key Point

High-pitched wheezing that occupies a large part of the respiratory cycle indicates severe airway obstruction.

The number of wheezes helps assess the extent of disease because each wheeze indicates partial obstruction of a bronchus. Single (or localized) wheezes indicate a localized area of narrowing (e.g., airway tumor), whereas multiple (generalized) wheezes indicate more widespread disorders, such as asthma or bronchitis.

Identifying the anatomical position where wheezing is loudest will also help indicate the origin. Wheezing that transmits to the mouth generally indicates that larger airways are involved, whereas wheezing heard only over the peripheral chest is probably the result of obstruction in more peripheral airways. Wheezing may be heard only over the trachea in some patients with asthma. When wheezing is only heard—or is heard predominately—over the upper sternum and supraglottic area, laryngeal dysfunction syndrome with inappropriate narrowing of the laryngeal area may be the cause. Wheezing heard only over one lung suggests mucus plugging or foreign body (such as a peanut) partially obstructing a large bronchus in the underlying lung.

The long-term implications of wheezing in infants has been studied. Infants who wheeze typically have transient conditions and are not at greater risk for asthma later in life.[23]

Paradoxical Absence of Wheezing. The absence of wheezing in a patient who previously was wheezing can be indicative of severe airway obstruction resulting in ventilatory failure. Rapid airflow past the site of obstruction is needed to set the airway walls in motion and create the musical sound. As the patient tires, the respiratory effort may diminish and result in less intense wheezing or no wheezing at all. This can be interpreted falsely as improvement if other clinical parameters are not assessed simultaneously. Evaluation of multiple clinical parameters, such as pulse, blood pressure, and patient orientation (along with the lung sounds), always provides a more accurate assessment than simply looking at any one parameter.

Therapeutic Implications of Wheezing. Wheezing is a common clinical sign of obstructive airway disease. With intrathoracic obstructive defects, wheezing is often expiratory but may be heard throughout the respiratory cycle. Multiple monophonic or polyphonic wheezing is a clinical sign of widespread airway obstruction, as seen with asthma or bronchitis. Bronchodilator therapy is indicated in such cases. The intensity of the wheeze does not indicate the degree of bronchodilator response to be expected. COPD patients who wheeze are more likely to have a significant response to bronchodilators and corticosteroids than those who do not wheeze.[24]

Airway secretions may contribute to the sound production process when the wheezing varies with coughing. Teaching the patient how to cough effectively and applying therapies to remove the excess secretions (e.g., aerosol treatments, postural drainage) can be helpful.

Therapy that improves the airway caliber should cause changes in the characteristics of the continuous adventitious lung sounds. The wheezing may decrease in pitch, duration, and intensity as airway obstruction diminishes. If treatment is effective, the wheezing may clear. The disappearance of wheezing can occur with ventilatory failure, as mentioned previously. Wheezing that does not respond to bronchodilators may be the result of laryngeal dysfunction syndrome, sometimes called *pseudoasthma*.

☞ Key Point

Polyphonic wheezing or multiple monophonic wheezes indicate the need for bronchodilator therapy.

Stridor

Most often, stridor is an inspiratory sound that is loud and can be heard at a distance from the patient. It indicates that partial laryngeal or tracheal obstruction is present. Epiglottitis, viral croup, foreign body aspiration, airway inflammation after extubation, tumors, vocal cord paralysis, laryngeal subglottic stenosis, and tracheal stenosis can cause stridor. Stridor occurs in about 15% of extubated patients and is more likely in those who have a difficult extubation.[25]

Stridor can be a sign of a potentially serious and life-threatening problem, especially in children. The patient with stridor must be closely watched and evaluated for signs of severe obstruction. As the obstruction worsens, stridor may become inspiratory and expiratory. The patient will begin using the accessory muscles to move air past the obstruction. Paradoxical pulse may occur. The presence of cyanosis in a patient with upper airway obstruction is a particularly ominous, troublesome sign. It indicates that airway obstruction is severe enough to cause ventilatory failure and hypoxemia.

Stridor may respond to cool mist and inhalation of racemic epinephrine in some cases. This treatment has proven beneficial in patients with airway inflammation due to laryngotracheobronchitis and after extubation. In all patients with stridor, however, close monitoring of the patient is critical, and the possible need to place an artificial airway must be considered in advance. In patients with dyspnea and a history suggestive of upper airway abnormality, the absence of stridor should not be interpreted to indicate normal airway patency.

☞ Key Point

> Stridor indicates narrowing of the upper airway and can be a sign of a life-threatening emergency. The patient with stridor should never be left alone and may need an artificial airway.

VOICE SOUNDS

Vocal resonance is created as the vibrations of phonation travel down the tracheobronchial tree and throughout the lung parenchyma. A normal air-filled lung transmits low-frequency sounds (<200 Hz), but higher frequencies are selectively filtered and attenuated. As a result, speech heard through a stethoscope over a normal lung is heard as a low-pitched mumble. Alteration in lung pathology will change the transmission of voice sounds, thus resulting in either increased or decreased transmission of vocal resonance.

An increase in vocal resonance, known as **bronchophony,** results in louder and clearer voice sounds over the affected area. This occurs with increases in lung tissue density, as in lung consolidation from pneumonia or atelectasis. In such cases, the acoustical filtering ability of the lung is reduced. Bronchophony is easier to detect when it is unilateral and is associated with bronchial breath sounds.

A reduction in vocal resonance occurs when lung tissue density decreases, thus resulting in more attenuaton of sound. This is typically identified with pulmonary hyperinflation disorders (e.g., emphysema, acute asthma) and is bilateral in such cases. Decreased vocal resonance is also noted over areas of the lung separated from the chest wall by pneumothorax or pleural effusion. The decrease in vocal resonance heard over pleural effusion or pneumothorax may be explained by reduced ventilation of the underlying lobe and/or by reflection of the sound (see Chapter 3).

When the voice sound increases in intensity and takes on a nasal or "bleating" quality, it is described as **egophony.** Egophony generally is identified over areas of the chest where bronchophony is present. The exact reason for this change in the voice sound is unknown. It is identified by asking the patient to say "e-e-e." If egophony is present, the "e-e-e" will be heard as "a-a-a" over the peripheral chest wall with a stethoscope. This most often is identified over consolidated lung, such as over an area of lobar pneumonia or an area of compressed lung above a pleural effusion.

Whispering creates high-frequency vibrations that are filtered out selectively by normal lung and normally heard as muffled, low-pitched sounds over the chest wall. When consolidation is present, however, the lung loses its selective transmitter quality, and the whispering is transmitted to the chest wall with more clarity. This sign, known as **whispered pectoriloquy,** is especially helpful to identify small or patchy areas of lung consolidation where more obvious signs may be absent. It is usually elicited by having the patient whisper "1-2-3" or "99."

As a result of modern technology, the use of voice sounds to assess the pulmonary patient is not as popular today as it was many years ago. The development of chest x-rays, CAT scans, and other technology has caused a shift away from the simple techniques of assessment to those that provide more objective information. Although this shift has proven expensive, in some cases it can be life-saving. This does not suggest that the simple techniques of assessment, such as evaluation of voice sounds, are a waste of time. Clinicians need to be aware of the evaluation options available to them in any given case and make a judgment call as to what techniques to employ.

☞ Key Point

Lung abnormalities that increase lung density often cause the voice sounds to become clearer and louder at the chest wall. The opposite is true for abnormalities that cause the lung density to decrease.

MISCELLANEOUS SOUNDS

In patients with chest hair, a crackling noise may be heard from the chest hair rubbing on the diaphragm of the stethoscope. Wetting the hair or pressing the stethoscope firmly to the skin will help to eliminate this extraneous sound. When air is present in the subcutaneous tissue (as with subcutaneous emphysema), a crackling noise can be heard when the stethoscope is pressed down over the affected area. When air is present in the mediastinum (pneumomediastinum) and sometimes with a left pneumothorax, a crunching or crackling sound may be heard with each heart beat and is called a *systolic* or **xiphi-sternal crunch.** If the patient has fractured ribs or a fractured sternum, the ends of the bone may rub against one another and cause a clicking sound. This is called **bone crepitus.** If water is present in the tubing between a mechanical ventilator and an endotracheal or tracheostomy tube, a gurgling or bubbling sound might be confused with coarse crackles when one is listening over the chest with a stethoscope.

Chapter Highlights

- Normal breath sounds can be categorized into four general types: tracheal, bronchial, bronchovesicular, and vesicular.
- There is no uniform agreement as to the origin of breath sounds, but most clinicians believe that inspiratory sounds are produced in the lung (not in the upper airways or the alveoli, but somewhere inbetween), whereas the expiratory phase is produced more centrally.
- When the vesicular breath sound increases in intensity, it is described as harsh, tubular, or tracheobronchial. This occurs when the attenuation properties of the lung parenchyma are reduced with consolidation.
- Diminished breath sounds result when the attenuation effect of the lung is increased, as with emphysema. A hyperinflated lung transmits sound poorly.
- Adventitious lung sounds (ALS) are abnormal sounds superimposed on the breath sounds. They are divided into continuous and discontinuous types.
- The recommended term for continuous ALS is *wheezes* and, for discontinuous ALS, *crackles.*
- Discontinuous adventitious lung sounds are produced by the sudden opening of collapsed airways or by the movement of air through excessive airway secretions.
- Continuous adventitious lung sounds are most often the result of airway obstruction that causes rapid airflow through the obstructed site, with resulting airway wall vibration.
- Fine, late-inspiratory crackles occur with restrictive lung disorders such as pulmonary fibrosis and atelectasis.
- Early-inspiratory crackles are common in patients with COPD. They are typically scanty and radiate to the mouth.
- Wheezing that is high pitched and occupies a large portion of the respiratory cycle (e.g., panexpiratory) is consistent with severe airway obstruction.
- Stridor is a sign of upper airway obstruction.
- The absence of wheezing or stridor in a patient with dyspnea may represent respiratory muscle fatigue.

REFERENCES

1. Kraman SS: Vesicular (normal) lung sounds: how are they made, where do they come from, and what do they mean? *Sem Resp Med* 6:183, 1985.
2. Pasterkamp H, Patel S, Wodicka GR: Asymmetry of respiratory sounds and thoracic transmission, *Med Biol Eng Comput* 35:103-106, 1997.
3. Bohadana AB, Peslin R, Uffholtz H: Breath sounds in the clinical assessment of airflow obstruction, *Thorax* 33:345, 1978.
4. Pardee NE, Martin CJ, Morgan EH: A test of the practical value of estimating breath sound intensity, *Chest* 70:341, 1976.
5. Kramin SS: The relationship between airflow and lung sound amplitude in normal subjects, *Chest* 86:225, 1984.
6. Ploysongsang Y, Iyer VK, Ramamoorthy PA: Reproducibility of the vesicular breath sounds in normal subjects, *Respiration* 58:158-162, 1991.
7. Mahagnah M, Gavriely N: Repeatability of measurements of normal lung sounds, *Am J Respir Crit Care Med* 149:477-481, 1994.
8. Heckerling PS: The need for chest roentgenograms in adults with acute respiratory illness, *Arch Intern Med* 146:1321, 1986.
9. Wilkins RL, Dexter JR: Comparing RCPs to physicians for the description of lung sounds: are we accurate and can we communicate? *Resp Care* 35:969-976, 1990.
10. Wilkins RL, Dexter JR, Murphy RLH, et al: Lung sounds nomenclature survey, *Chest* 98:886-889, 1990.
11. Mikami R, Murao M, Cugell DW: International symposium on lung sounds, *Chest* 92:342-345, 1987.
12. Robertson AJ, Coope R: Rales, rhonchi, and Laennec, *Lancet* 2:417-423, 1957.
13. Wilkins RL, Dexter JR, Smith MP, et al: Lung sound terminology used by respiratory care practitioners, *Resp Care* 34:36-41, 1989.
14. Al Jarad N, Davies SW, Logan-Sinclair R, et al: Lung crackle characteristics in patients with asbestosis, asbestos-related pleural disease and left ventricular failure using a time-expanded waveform analysis: a comparative study, *Resp Med* 88:37-46, 1994.
15. Baughman RP, Shipley RT, Loudon RG, et al: Crackles in interstitial lung disease, *Chest* 100:96-101, 1991.
16. Bettencourt PE et al: Clinical utility of chest auscultation in common pulmonar diseases, *Am J Respir Crit Care Med* 150:1291-1297, 1994.
17. Nath AR, Capel LH: Lung crackles in bronchiectasis, *Thorax* 35:694, 1980.
18. Thacker RE, Kraman SS: The prevalence of auscultatory crackles in subjects without lung disease, *Chest* 81:672, 1982.
19. Kiyokawa H, Greenberg M, Shirota K, et al: Auditory detection of simulated crackles in breath sounds, *Chest* 119:1886-1892, 2001.
20. Braughman RP, Loudon RG: Quantification of wheezing in acute asthma, *Chest* 86:718, 1984.

21. Braughman RP, Loudon RG: Stridor: differentiation from asthma or upper airway noise, *Am Rev Respir Dis* 139:1407-1409, 1989.
22. Braughman RP, Loudon RG: Lung sound analysis for continuous evaluation of airflow obstruction in asthma, *Chest* 88:364, 1985.
23. Martinez FD et al: Asthma and wheezing in the first six years of life, *N Engl J Med* 332:133-138, 1995.
24. Marini JJ, Pierson DJ, Hudson LD, et al: The significance of wheezing in chronic airflow obstruction, *Am Rev Resp Dis* 120:1069, 1979.
25. Jaber S: Postextubation stridor in intensive care patients: risk factors, evaluation and importance of cuff-leak test. *Intensive Care Med* 29:69-74, 2003.

Review Questions

1. Which of the following breath sounds is normally lowest in pitch?
   A. Tracheal
   B. Bronchial
   C. Bronchovesicular
   D. Vesicular

2. Which of the following breath sounds has a pause between the inspiratory and the expiratory component?
   A. Tracheal
   B. Bronchial
   C. Bronchovesicular
   D. Vesicular

3. Which of the following terms is *not* appropriate to describe harsh breath sounds heard over the peripheral chest that have an equal inspiratory and expiratory component?
   A. Tubular
   B. Bronchial
   C. Tracheobronchial
   D. Vesicular

4. True or False
   The normal breath sounds are produced regionally within each lung and probably within each lobe.

5. Which of the following conditions increases the attenuation properties of the lung?
   A. Pneumonia
   B. Emphysema
   C. Pleural effusion
   D. B and C

Review Questions—cont'd

6. Your patient has reduced breath sounds over a specific lobe. Which of the following conditions is *not* likely to be the cause?
   A. Mucus plugging
   B. Bronchial intubation
   C. Pulmonary fibrosis
   D. Bronchial obstruction

7. What therapy may be helpful to treat the patient with bronchial breath sounds over the dependent regions?
   A. Lung expansion therapy
   B. Postural drainage
   C. Aerosol therapy
   D. All of the above

8. Continuous adventitious lung sounds are *best* described with what term?
   A. Rhonchi
   B. Rales
   C. Crackles
   D. Wheezes

9. Discontinuous adventitious lung sounds are *best* described with what term?
   A. Rhonchi
   B. Rales
   C. Crackles
   D. Wheezes

10. Which of the following qualifying adjectives is *least* appropriate?
    A. Fine
    B. Medium
    C. Sibilant
    D. High-pitched

11. Which of the following conditions is *not* likely to produce fine, late-inspiratory crackles?
    A. Atelectasis
    B. Pleural effusion
    C. Pulmonary fibrosis
    D. Congestive heart failure

12. Which of the following is associated with continuous ALS?
    A. Narrowing of intrathoracic airways
    B. Narrowing of extrathoracic airway
    C. Fixed extrathoracic obstruction
    D. All of the above

Continued

Review Questions—cont'd

13. What therapy is indicated for the patient with late-inspiratory crackles?
   A. Incentive spirometry
   B. Oxygen
   C. Mucolytics
   D. Bronchodilators

14. Which of the following may decrease when bronchodilator therapy is effective in treating wheezing?
   A. The pitch of the wheeze
   B. The portion of the respiratory cycle occupied by the wheeze
   C. The intensity of the wheeze
   D. All of the above

15. Monophonic wheezing heard over a single lobe is suggestive of what possible problem?
   A. Asthma
   B. Bronchitis
   C. Emphysema
   D. Foreign body aspiration

16. About what percent of patients have stridor after extubation?
   A. 15%
   B. 30%
   C. 45%
   D. 60%

17. Which of the following treatments is *most* useful for the treatment of the patient with stridor as a result of upper airway inflammation?
   A. Bronchodilators
   B. Cool mist and racemic epinephrine
   C. Postural drainage
   D. CPAP

18. Which of the following may cause an increase in vocal resonance?
   A. Atelectasis
   B. Pneumonia
   C. Asthma
   D. A and B

19. Which of the following is associated with a decrease in vocal resonance?
   A. Emphysema
   B. Pneumonia
   C. Atelectasis
   D. None of the above

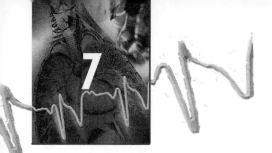

Heart Sounds

OBJECTIVES

After reading this chapter, you will be able to recognize and describe the following:
- The appropriate terms used to describe normal and abnormal heart sounds.
- The mechanisms responsible for the production of normal and abnormal heart sounds.
- The correct interpretation of the findings during cardiac auscultation.

KEY TERMS

gallop rhythm	physiologic murmur	S4
murmurs	S1	split S1
pericardial friction	S2	split S2
rub	S3	

R ecognizing and interpreting heart sounds represents a significant challenge for health care providers. The sounds of the heart are often very faint even when normal, and abnormalities can be very subtle. Only through comprehension of cardiac anatomy (see Chapter 2) and a clear understanding of how heart sounds are created can the clinician use the clues provided during cardiac auscultation to make proper clinical decisions. The purpose of this chapter is to provide the reader with information about how heart sounds are created and how the findings are to be interpreted.

TERMINOLOGY AND MECHANISMS

S1 and S2

The terms used to document heart sounds have not had a controversial history like those used to document lung sounds. The normal beating heart has a basic first and second heart sound with each cardiac cycle.

Table 7-1	Assessing the Heart Sounds		
Sound	Location	Chestpiece	Mechanism
S1	Apex	Diaphragm	Closure of the A-V valves
S2	Base	Diaphragm	Closure of the semilunar valves
S3	Apex	Bell	Passive filling of the ventricles
S4	Apex	Bell	Active filling of the ventricles

The initial sound is called **S1;** the second sound is **S2.** S1 is produced by closure of the atrial-ventricular (A-V) valves (mitral and tricuspid) during ventricular systole. The A-V valves close when ventricular pressure rapidly increases during systole and causes the ventricular pressure to exceed the pressure in the atria. S1 is best heard over the apex of the heart but is heard over the entire precordium in most patients. Because left-sided pressures are greater than right-sided pressures, the mitral valve component (M1) is louder than the tricuspid valve component (T1) normally. S1 is a high-frequency sound best heard with the diaphragm portion of the stethoscope (Table 7-1).

S2 is produced by closure of the semilunar valves (aortic and pulmonic) during ventricular diastole. These valves close when the pressure in the ventricles drops during diastole and the pressure in the aorta and pulmonary artery exceed ventricular diastolic pressure. S2 is best heard over the base of the heart. Because the left side of the heart generates greater pressures, the aortic component (A2) is louder than the pulmonic component (P2) normally. Because both components of S2 are high-frequency sounds, S2 is best heard with the diaphragm portion of the stethoscope (see Table 7-1).

The main heart sounds just described, S1 and S2, provide reference points that help time and describe the abnormal sounds discussed below.

☞ Key Point

The first heart sound (S1) is produced by closure of the A-V valves. The second heart sound (S2) is produced by closure of the semilunar valves.

S3 and S4

In some healthy people and in many with heart disease, a third **(S3)** and/or fourth heart sound **(S4)** may be present. S3 is produced early in diastole (immediately after S2) when the A-V valves initially open and the blood collecting in the atria passively enters the ventricles and

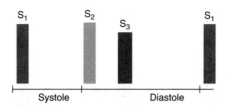

Figure 7-1. S3, an early diastolic sound. *(From Barkauskas VH, Baumann LC, Darling-Fisher CS: Health and physical assessment, ed 3, St Louis, 2002, Mosby.)*

contacts the ventricular walls, causing them to vibrate temporarily. S3 can occur in healthy young people when cardiac output is elevated and ventricular filling is rapid and more forceful. It is called *physiologic S3* in such cases. Most often it occurs in those with heart disease when the ventricular wall is abnormal, as occurs after a myocardial infarction and is commonly indicative of congestive heart failure. The ventricular wall in such cases is stiffer than normal and the lack of compliance leads to a thumping type of noise when a bolus of blood makes contact. S3 is a dull, low-pitched sound best heard with the bell over the apex (see Table 7-1).

S4 is produced in a similar way as S3 but occurs late in diastole (just before S1) when the atria contract and actively send a bolus of blood into the ventricles just before systole. S4 also is a dull, low-pitched sound best heard with the bell. S4 may occur, similar to S3, in healthy people in high cardiac output settings but is more often heard in patients with an abnormal left ventricle. A loud S4 always suggests pathology and more investigation is needed. The only difference between S4 and S3 is the timing in which the sound is heard during diastole (Figures 7-1 and 7-2). It is possible for someone to have an S3 without an S4 and likewise an S4 could be present without an S3. In addition, it is possible for both to be present. S3s and S4s are quiet sounds that are difficult to hear in most cases. Increases in venous return will cause a temporary increase in the intensity of an S3 or S4 while decreases in venous return (as occurs with positive pressure

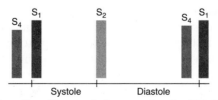

Figure 7-2. S4, a late diastolic sound. *(From Barkauskas VH, Baumann LC, Darling-Fisher CS: Health and physical assessment, ed 3, St Louis, 2002, Mosby.)*

ventilation) may cause the sounds to diminish. S4 is also best heard over the apex of the heart with the bell (see Table 7-1).

☞ Key Point

During diastole, filling of the ventricles may produce an added heart sound that may occur right after S2 and is called an S3 in such cases, or just before the subsequent S1 and is called an S4 in such cases.

Splitting of S1 and S2

Both S1 and S2 are each produced by closure of two separate valves. In certain circumstances, one side of the heart will not be in exact sequence with the other side of the heart. For example, if the left side of the heart contracts slightly ahead of the right side of the heart, the mitral valve will close slightly ahead of the tricuspid valve. This causes the first heart sound to have two distinct components and is known as a **split S1.** A split S1 almost always signifies an abnormality with the heart such as an electrical conduction defect (e.g., bundle branch block). It is difficult to hear because the tricuspid component of S1 is very faint due to the low pressures on the right side of the heart.

Splitting of S2 is more common and almost expected. A split of S2 is more common during inspiration as the drop in intrathoracic pressure that occurs during inspiration causes a temporary increase in right ventricular filling and a slight delay in closure of the pulmonic valve. It is called a physiologic **split S2** in such cases and is most notable at peak inspiration and should disappear during expiration. Interpretation of split S1 and S2 is discussed later in this chapter.

Murmurs

Adventitious heart sounds are called **murmurs.** Murmurs are produced by the following:

1. Rapid bloodflow over a normal valve (**physiologic murmur**)
2. Bloodflow over a narrowed valve (Figure 7-3)
3. Backflow of blood through an incompetent valve
4. Bloodflow through an abnormal opening (e.g., ventricular septal defect)

The most common cause of murmurs is a faulty heart valve. Stenotic heart valves represent incomplete opening of the valve and cause murmurs when blood passes through the narrowed opening, especially when blood flow is rapid. Stenosis of a semilunar valve causes a systolic murmur and stenosis of an A-V valve causes a diastolic murmur. Thus the timing of the murmur plays an important role in determining the location and type of the defect.

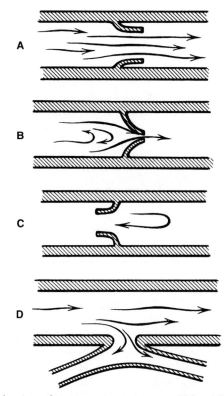

Figure 7-3. Mechanisms for murmurs. **A,** Increased blood flow across a normal valve; **B,** forward flow through a stenotic valve; **C,** backflow (regurgitation) through an incompetent valve; and **D,** flow through an abnormal opening, such as a septal defect or an arteriovenous fistula (patent ductus arteriosus). *(From Barkauskas VH, Baumann LC, Darling-Fisher CS:* Health and physical assessment, *ed 3, St Louis, 2002, Mosby.)*

In addition to becoming stenotic, heart valves may become incompetent and not seat properly when they close. This causes regurgitation of blood back into the chamber from where it came and will cause a murmur. An incompetent A-V valve will cause a systolic murmur, and an incompetent semilunar valve will cause a diastolic murmur.

In addition to timing during the cardiac cycle, another important factor to consider when evaluating a patient with a murmur is the exact location on the precordium where the murmur is best heard. Because each heart valve has a specific location on the chest wall where it may best be heard (see Chapter 4), this can prove useful in identifying the defective valve when a murmur is present. For example, if a systolic murmur is present and it is loudest at the second right intercostal space at the sternal border (the aortic valve area [see Chapter 4]), a stenotic aortic valve is likely to be the cause.

☞ Key Point

Adventitious heart sounds are called *murmurs*. They are produced by blood flow passing forward through a narrowed opening or backward through an incompetent valve. Systolic murmurs may be physiologic in young healthy people but usually represent an abnormal heart valve in older patients. Diastolic murmurs are always abnormal and representative of valve incompetence or stenosis.

INTERPRETATION OF HEART SOUNDS

S1 and S2

The primary feature of the basic heart sounds to identify is their intensity. S1 and S2 can be normal, soft, or loud. The beginner may have difficulty in determining changes in the heart sound intensity as these changes are often subtle. As with breath sounds, the heart sounds can be present in normal intensity but difficult to hear because of attenuation of sound through the chest wall. For example, an obese patient or one with a muscular chest wall may have a healthy heart but the heart sounds will appear distant because of attenuation. In addition, pulmonary hyperinflation, such as occurs with emphysema, can cause significant problems with transmission of the heart sounds through the chest wall. In patients with severe hyperinflation, the heart sounds, rate, and rhythm are best detected by listening with the stethoscope positioned in the epigastrium.

Diminished heart sounds can occur as a result of pathologic or physiologic changes in the heart. S1 can be diminished when the leaflets of the valves are rigid and not mobile. Rigid heart valves (e.g., mitral stenosis) do not close sharply and produce diminished heart sounds. The position of the valve leaflets just before systole can also play a role in a diminished S1. For example, if the heart rate is particularly slow, filling of the ventricles will be more complete and the valve leaflets will "float" to a more closed position before systole. This results in a softer S1 since the valve leaflets have little distance to travel once ventricular systole occurs. Finally, S1 can be diminished with reduced contractility of the heart. This is common following a myocardial infarction or as a side effect of some medications (e.g., beta blockers).

Diminished S2 occurs when the pressures in the aorta and/or pulmonary artery are reduced. This may be present with severe hypovolemia or with systemic hypotension as occurs in shock. Stenosis of the aortic valve also can cause a diminished S2.

☞ Key Point

S1 and S2 are evaluated for their intensity. Decreased or soft heart sounds are the result of poor contractility or stenotic valves that do not snap closed. Increased attenuation of the heart sounds occurs with obesity and severe pulmonary hyperinflation.

Increases in the intensity of S1 can occur for a variety of reasons. Faster heart rates often cause a louder S1 as the leaflets of the A-V valves are wide apart with the onset of systole and the valves are "slammed" shut in such cases. Increased contractility will lead to a louder S1 and is seen with exercise and other high cardiac output situations (e.g., anemia, high fever, etc.).

A loud S2 is common when the pressure in the aorta is higher than normal, as occurs with systemic hypertension. Elevation of the diastolic pressure causes the aortic valve to be forced closed with each diastole. Elevation of the pressure in the pulmonary artery causes the pulmonic valve to be closed with increased force, and this may be heard as a loud S2. When a loud S2 is present, the examiner should listen specifically to the aortic and pulmonic areas on the chest wall (see Chapter 4). A *loud P2* is said to be present when the S2 is louder over the pulmonic area. Pulmonary hypertension is probably the cause in such cases. A loud A2 is present when the increase in S2 is best heard over the aortic area on the chest wall and is consistent with systemic hypertension. Splitting of S2 is common when a loud P2 or A2 is present. With a loud P2, the second component of the split S2 will be louder than normal. With a loud A2, the first component will be louder than normal.

☞ Key Point

A loud P2 is a sign of pulmonary hypertension. It is a clue that the patient may suffer from chronic lung disease, chronic left ventricular dysfunction, pulmonary embolism, or primary pulmonary hypertension.

Split S1 and S2

Splitting of the heart sounds that is not physiologic can be *wide, fixed,* or *paradoxic* (Figure 7-4). Wide splitting refers to a more noticeable delay between the two components of S1 and/or S2. This is common

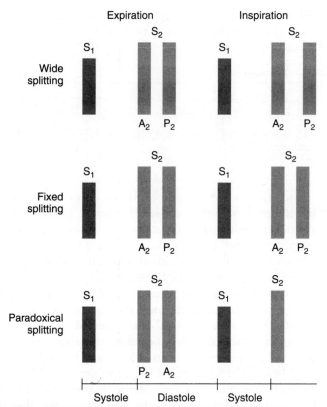

Figure 7-4. Variations in splitting of S2. *(From Seidel HM, Ball JW, Dains JE, et al: Mosby's guide to physical examination, ed 5, St Louis, 2003, Mosby.)*

when the electrical conduction system of the heart is damaged, as in right bundle branch block. In such cases, both S1 and S2 will have a wide split as the left side of the heart is significantly ahead of the right side (see Figure 7-4). Closure of the mitral and aortic valves will occur before closure of the tricuspid and pulmonic valves, respectively, during the cardiac cycle. Wide splitting of S2 is common with pulmonary hypertension when closure of the pulmonic valve is delayed because of slow emptying of the right ventricle as a result of high right ventricular afterload.

Fixed splitting of S2 is present when the splitting does not alter with respiration. It occurs most often when the pulmonic valve is delayed in closing because the output of the right ventricle is significantly greater than that of the left ventricle. This is common in large atrial septal defects and ventricular septal defects with left to right shunting. Right ventricular failure also can cause fixed splitting of S2.

Paradoxic splitting is present when P2 occurs before A2. This is most often the result of left bundle branch block. Respiration will alter the splitting in this situation, with the splitting increasing during expiration and decreasing during inspiration.

S3 and S4

The presence of an S3 and/or S4 results in a heart rhythm that resembles the sound made by the gallop of a horse. For this reason, patients with these added heart sounds are said to have a **gallop rhythm.** Gallop rhythms are common in patients with heart disease and suggest volume overload as occurs in congestive heart failure or a noncompliant ventricle, as seen in myocardial infarction or with ventricular hypertrophy. Advanced mitral or tricuspid valve regurgitation also can result in a gallop rhythm. Chronic drug or alcohol abuse can cause cardiomyopathy (disease of the myocardium) and result in ventricular hypertrophy and a gallop rhythm.

☞ Key Point

A gallop rhythm in patients over 40 years of age signifies heart disease. The patient should be evaluated for left ventricular failure or recent myocardial infarction.

Murmurs

Murmurs are evaluated for intensity, pitch, timing, and location. These variables help the clinician interpret the underlying pathology responsible for the murmur.

Murmurs are typically graded on a scale of I to VI based on intensity. Grade I murmurs are very soft and may only be heard by a well-trained cardiologist with a quality stethoscope in a quiet room (Table 7-2). Each step up in the grading system represents a slightly louder murmur and eventually ends in a grade VI murmur that can be heard

Table 7-2 | Grading Murmurs

Grade I	Barely audible in a quiet room with a good stethoscope
Grade II	Soft but audible
Grade III	Moderately loud
Grade IV	Loud and associated with a thrill
Grade V	Very loud and associated with a thrill that is easily palpable
Grade VI	Very loud and can be heard with a stethoscope not in contact with the patient's chest

without the aid of a stethoscope against the chest. The grade of a murmur may not correlate with any degree of pathology because intensity is a function of interaction between degree of narrowing and speed of blood flow.

Systolic ejection murmurs occur when blood flow out of one of the ventricles is impeded by a narrowed semilunar valve. Aortic stenosis will produce a medium-pitched, midsystolic murmur that has a crescendo-decrescendo quality heard loudest at the second right inter-costal space. The systolic ejection murmur-related stenosis of the aortic valve commonly radiates to the carotid arteries in the neck. Pulmonic stenosis produces a similar murmur that is best heard at the second left intercostal space. The murmur associated with stenosis of the pulmonic valve will often be louder on inspiration due to the increased blood flow to the right side of the heart associated with a drop in intrathoracic pressure.

Systolic murmurs can also occur when regurgitation occurs because of incompetence of the mitral or tricuspid valves. The murmur will be pansystolic and have a soft blowing quality in such cases (Table 7-3). Tricuspid regurgitation murmurs are affected by breathing (increase with inspiration), whereas mitral valve regurgitation murmurs are not. Murmurs due to mitral valve regurgitation or incompetence are heard at the apex of the heart and commonly radiate to the left mid-axillary line. Systolic regurgitation murmurs are best heard with the diaphragm portion of the chestpiece.

☞ Key Point

Midsystolic murmurs are associated with stenosis of a semilunar valve. Pansystolic murmurs are associated with incompetence of an A-V valve.

An atrial or ventricular septal defect will also produce a systolic mur-mur. An atrial septal defect causes increased blood flow through the

Table 7-3	Assessing Heart Murmurs		
Murmur type	Timing	Quality	Mechanism
Systolic	Mid	Medium pitched	Stenosis of semilunar valves
Systolic	Pan	Soft blowing	Incompetence of A-V valves
Diastolic	Mid to late	Low pitched	Stenosis of A-V valves
Diastolic	Early	Decrescendo	Incompetence of semilunar valves

pulmonic valve (because of left to right shunting), which results in the murmur. Murmurs due to atrial septal defects are best heard over the base of the heart. Ventricular septal defects cause a murmur because of the shunting of blood through the defect from the left ventricle to the right ventricle and may also cause a murmur associated with increased blood flow through the pulmonic valve. Ventricular septal defect murmurs are best heard at the apex of the heart. With long-standing left to right shunts through septal defects, pulmonary hypertension may develop, thus leading to a reversal of the flow of blood from right to left through the septal defect.

Diastolic murmurs occur when the A-V valves are stenotic or when the semilunar valves are incompetent. Stenotic A-V valves cause mid to late diastolic murmurs that are best heard with the bell portion of the chestpiece because they are low-pitched sounds. They are best heard over the apex of the heart. Incompetent semilunar valves cause murmurs because of regurgitation of the blood back into the ventricle of the involved side during diastole. These types of murmurs are present early in diastole and are best heard with the diaphragm portion of the chestpiece. They are described as high-pitched decrescendo murmurs. They are loudest over the base of the heart. The low-pitched diastolic rumble of mitral valve stenosis is generally heard best at the apex with the patient laying on his or her left side. The early diastolic murmur of aortic valve regurgitation is often heard best to the left of the sternum with the patient sitting up and leaning forward.

✍ Key Point

Diastolic murmurs that are mid to late in diastole are usually caused by stenotic A-V valves. Incompetent semilunar valves cause murmurs early in diastole.

Pericardial Friction Rub

A **pericardial friction rub** may be heard when the pericardial sac becomes inflamed. Inflammation of this sac produces a grating sound as the heart beats inside the sac. The sound is similar to that heard with a pleural friction rub during lung auscultation (see Chapter 6). Pericardial friction rubs are best heard over the apex of the heart and may make it difficult to hear S1 and S2.

Chapter Highlights

- The first heart sound is produced by closure of the A-V valves during systole and is called *S1*.
- The second heart sound is produced by closure of the semilunar valves during diastole and is called *S2*.
- In some patients, extra heart sounds may be present and are referred to as S3 and S4. They are produced by rapid filling of the ventricles during diastole. S3 occurs early in diastole from passive filling and S4 late in diastole from active filling (atrial contraction).
- A gallop rhythm is said to be present when an S3 or S4 or both are present. It usually signifies left ventricular hypertrophy, myocardial infarction, or congestive heart failure.
- Splitting of S1 is present when the mitral and tricuspid valves do not close simultaneously. This is seen in bundle branch block.
- Splitting of S2 occurs in healthy people because of the effects of breathing on venous return to the heart. It is called a *physiologic split* in such cases. Disorders of the heart may also cause splitting of S2 and cause it to become wide, fixed, or paradoxic.
- Murmurs are adventitious heart sounds that are produced most often from forward blood flow through a narrowed (stenotic) valve or with backflow through an incompetent valve.
- Systolic murmurs are produced when the semilunar valves are stenotic or when the A-V valves are incompetent.
- Diastolic murmurs occur when the A-V valves are stenotic or when the semilunar valves are incompetent.
- An ejection midsystolic murmur is consistent with stenosis of the aortic or pulmonic valve.
- A pansystolic murmur indicates regurgitation of blood from the left or right ventricle into the respective atrium due to a faulty A-V valve.
- A low-pitched, rumbling, mid to late diastolic murmur is consistent with a stenotic A-V valve.
- An early, decrescendo diastolic murmur suggests an incompetent semilunar valve.
- Inflammation of the pericardial sac can cause a grating sound to occur with ventricular systole and diastole. This sound is called a pericardial friction rub.

BIBLIOGRAPHY

- Barkauskas VH, Baumann LC, Darling-Fisher CS: *Health and physical assessment*, ed 3, St Louis, 2002, Mosby.
- Lilly LS: *Pathophysiology of heart disease*, ed 3, Philadelphia, 2003, Lippincott, Williams and Wilkins.
- Seidel HM, Ball JW, Dains JE, et al: *Mosby's guide to physical examination*, ed 5, St Louis, 2003, Mosby.

Review Questions

1. True or False

S1 is produced by closure of the semilunar valves.

2. True or False

S1 is best heard over the apex of the heart.

3. True or False

S1 is best heard with the bell portion of the chestpiece.

4. True or False

Normally the aortic component (A2) is louder than the pulmonic component (P2) in producing the second heart sound.

5. True or False

An S3 is produced by filling of the left ventricle during diastole in patients with an abnormal left ventricle in most cases.

6. True or False

The only difference between an S3 and an S4 is the timing of the sound.

7. True or False

A loud S4 may not indicate disease in all cases.

8. True or False

Splitting of S2 is more common than splitting of S1.

9. Which of the following is *not* a common cause of diminished heart sounds?

    A. Rigid leaflets of the heart valves

    B. Slow heart rate

    C. Reduced contractility

    D. The use of bronchodilators

10. Which of the following causes a loud S2?

    A. Systemic hypertension

    B. Use of vasodilators

    C. Decreased contractility

    D. Fast heart rate

11. What is a common cause of a loud P2?

    A. Systemic hypertension

    B. Pulmonary hypertension

    C. High cardiac output

    D. Increased contractility

Continued

Review Questions—cont'd

12. Which of the following causes wide splitting of S2?
A. Systemic hypertension
B. Pulmonary hypertension
C. Use of vasodilators
D. Reduced cardiac output

13. What is a common cause of a gallop rhythm?
A. Asthma
B. Mitral stenosis
C. Congestive heart failure
D. Pericardial tamponade

14. Your patient has a pansystolic murmur with a soft blowing quality. What is the likely cause?
A. Mitral valve regurgitation
B. Aortic stenosis
C. Pulmonic stenosis
D. Tricuspid stenosis

15. Your patient has a diastolic murmur that is loudest over the base of the heart. It is described as a high-pitched decrescendo murmur. What problem is likely to be the cause?
A. Aortic valve regurgitation
B. Mitral valve stenosis
C. Tricuspid valve regurgitation
D. Mitral valve regurgitation

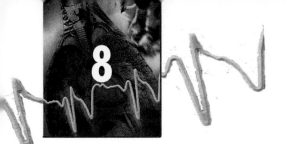

8

Case Studies

James R. Dexter, MD

This chapter provides 10 case studies as illustrations of how auscultation findings can be helpful in the assessment of patients with cardiopulmonary disease. In each case, the patient's history, physical examination findings, and other clinical data are presented to provide a clinical picture. Lung or heart sounds for each case example are presented on the accompanying audio program and should be reviewed as the chest examination findings are read. At the end of each case, several questions are listed to stimulate thinking. The answers to the questions are reviewed at the end of the chapter.

🕮 Case #1

History of Present Illness

A 36-year-old white female with exertional dyspnea that has gradually worsened over the last several years is seen in the outpatient clinic. Several years earlier, the patient had stopped jogging because of dyspnea. She now finds that her exercise tolerance is limited to walking one block or a half-flight of stairs. The patient denies cough, sputum production, wheezing, fever, night sweats, chest pain, orthopnea, or allergies. She knows of no aspirin sensitivity and has no sinus congestion.

Past Medical History

Illnesses: Unknown.

Familial Illnesses: Father died of emphysema at the age of 52, and one older brother has been told he has obstructive pulmonary disease.

Occupational History: Patient has worked as a checkout clerk at a local grocery store. No exposure to pulmonary toxins is known.

Pets: None.

Travel: Vacation in the southeastern United States 6 months ago.

Hobbies: Fishing.

Surgeries: None.

Marital Status: Single.

Medications: None.

TB History: No exposure; no skin tests.

Smoking History: 10 pack years; patient currently does not use tobacco.

Allergies: None.

Physical Examination

General: The patient is a well-nourished, well-developed white female in no acute distress at rest. Affect is appropriate.

Vital Signs: Within normal limits.

HEENT: Noncontributory to the present problem.

Neck: The trachea is midline and mobile. There is no stridor on tidal volume or forced vital capacity maneuvers. Carotid pulsations are normal and symmetrical. There are no carotid bruits and no lymphadenopathy. Accessory muscles are used for breathing with minimal exertion.

Chest: There is a substantially increased AP diameter, and there is decreased expansion with respiration. Increased resonance is noted upon percussion.

Heart: Cardiac sounds are mildly diminished. There is no right ventricular heave. The cardiac sounds are regular in rhythm without murmurs, gallops, or rubs.

Lungs: Refer to Case #1 on the audio program for the patient's lung sounds.

Abdomen: Soft and nontender. Bowel sounds are present. The liver is percussed 2 cm below the costal margin; however, the total width is only 10 cm at the midclavicular line.

Extremities: There is no cyanosis, clubbing, or edema. Pulses are +2 and symmetrical in all areas.

Lab Data

Chest Radiograph: See Figure 8-1.

Pulmonary Function Studies: $FEF_{25\%-75\%}$ is 28% of predicted, FVC is 84% of predicted, FEV_1 is 45% of predicted, and DLCO is 48% of predicted. No significant change after bronchodilator inhalation.

Questions for Case #1
1. Describe the breath sounds heard from Case #1 on the accompanying audio program.
2. What pulmonary disorders can cause this patient's problem?
3. What information supports the most likely diagnosis for this patient's problems over the other possibilities?
4. What is the most likely diagnosis?
5. What physiologic principles underlie the auscultatory findings in this case?
6. Are the breath sounds consistent with the pulmonary function test results?
7. What abnormalities are present on the chest radiograph?

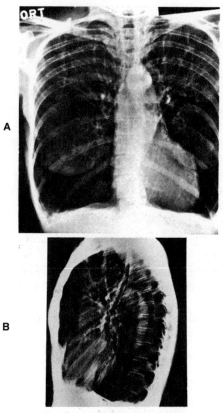

Figure 8-1. Radiographs of the chest in **A,** posteroanterior and **B,** lateral projections.

Case #2

History of Present Illness

The patient is a 38-year-old female with a 12-month history of wheezing, cough, and gradually increasing dyspnea on exertion (despite regular use of a large variety of medications including the following: inhaled beta agonists, inhaled steroids, and oral antibiotics). Other symptoms and signs include severe morning cough and daily sputum production of approximately $\frac{1}{4}$ cup of yellow to green mucus. Her cough has changed substantially over the past 6 months and is becoming more brassy in nature. Exercise tolerance is currently 2 to 3 blocks at a normal pace. Patient has noticed a 5-lb weight loss since the onset of her symptoms. Pertinent negative symptoms include the absence of chest pain, fevers, night sweats, orthopnea, and pedal edema.

Past Medical History

Illnesses: Childhood diseases include whooping cough, measles, and mumps.

Familial Illnesses: Father had TB in 1948 and coronary artery bypass graft in 1978. Mother and three siblings are well.

Occupational History: Realtor.

Pets: Bloodhound and goldfish.

Travel: Hawaiian holiday 4 months before the symptoms began.

Hobbies: Bridge and golf.

Surgeries: None.

Marital Status: Divorced for 10 years.

Medications: Metered-dose inhalers (salmeterol and fluticasone); prednisone (several courses of 40 mg per day, each course of 2 weeks' duration); antibiotics (short courses of 7–10 days trimethoprim/sulfamethoxazole, ampicillin, tetracycline, or erythromycin), without evidence of substantial improvement.

Smoking History: 30 pack years.

Allergies: Sensitivities to pollens and cats.

Physical Examination

General: The patient is a well-nourished, well-developed white female who appears slightly older than her stated age of 38. She is alert, oriented, and in no acute respiratory distress sitting in a chair.

Vital Signs: Within normal limits.

HEENT: Examination does not provide evidence contributory to the present problem.

Neck: The trachea is midline and mobile to palpation. There is no swelling of the lymph glands, no jugular venous distention, and no bruits heard over the carotid arteries. Carotid pulsations are symmetrical.

Chest: Normal AP diameter and normal expansion with breathing.

Heart: Regular rate and rhythm without murmurs, gallops, or rubs. No ventricular heaves.

Lungs: Refer to Case #2 on the accompanying audio program for example of the patient's breath sounds heard over the upper airway. Inspiratory and expiratory monophonic wheezing is heard over the upper lung fields. Faint monophonic wheezing is heard over the lower lobes.

Abdomen: Soft and nontender to palpations. No masses or organomegaly are noted. Bowel sounds are normal.

Extremities: There is no evidence of cyanosis, clubbing, or edema. Peripheral pulses are normal and bilaterally symmetrical.

Lab Data

ECG: Normal.

Pulmonary Function Tests: Flow-volume loops show marked reduction in inspiratory flow rates (Figure 8-2).

Chest Radiograph: Normal.

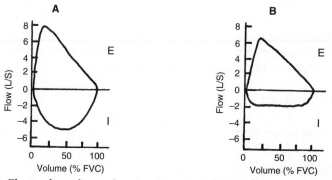

Figure 8-2. Flow-volume loops showing **A,** a normal individual and **B,** a patient with an extrathoracic large airway obstruction. Note the plateau representing limited inspiratory flow on the inspiratory loop in **B.** *I,* Inspiration; *E,* expiration.

Questions for Case #2

1. Describe the breath sounds heard on auscultation over the neck.
2. What pulmonary disorders can cause this patient's problem?
3. What information supports the most likely diagnosis for this patient's problems over the other possibilities?
4. What is the most likely diagnosis?
5. What physiologic principles underlie the auscultatory findings in this case?
6. What pathophysiology may explain the flow-volume loop results?
7. What procedure should be done next to diagnose the patient's problem?

Case #3

History of Present Illness

You are asked to evaluate a 35-year-old male who has been treated on the psychiatric ward of the hospital for approximately 30 days. He was without physical complaints until the afternoon of the request, when he noticed a sharp pain in his right chest and slight dyspnea while playing table tennis. The pain was of sudden onset, became worse with breathing, and improved when he held his breath. It radiated through to his back but not to his shoulder or jaw. It did not change with exercise or change in position. He has no other complaints and specifically denies a history of asthma, hay fever, and allergies. He also denies cough, fever, sputum production, night sweats, and orthopnea.

Past Medical History

Illnesses: Childhood diseases, including measles and mumps.

Familial Illnesses: Noncontributory.

Occupational History: Truck driver for a local egg company.

Pets: Staffordshire terrier.

Travel: Patient has not travelled outside of southern California.

Hobbies: Pool, table tennis, and dirt bike racing.

Surgeries: Appendectomy at age 12 and tonsillectomy at age 13.

Marital Status: Married with one child.

Medications: Lithium, effexor 300 mg/qd.

Smoking History: 45 pack years (started at age 12).

Allergies: Grass, penicillin, and stelazine.

Physical Examination

General: The patient is a tall, thin, white male who appears approximately his stated age of 35. He is alert, oriented, and in no respiratory distress while sitting up during the examination.

Vital Signs: Normal except for a pulse rate of 100/min.

HEENT: Examination does not provide evidence contributory to the pulmonary problem.

Neck: The trachea is mildly deviated toward the left but is mobile to palpation. There is no lymphadenopathy, jugular venous distention, or carotid bruits. Carotid pulsations are normal and symmetrical bilaterally.

Chest: The chest is asymmetrical, and there is more movement on the left side with breathing. Percussion of the chest reveals increased resonance over the right chest.

Heart: Regular rate and rhythm without murmurs, gallops, or rubs. No ventricular heaves are noted.

Lungs: Refer to Case #3 on the accompanying audio program for the patient's lung sounds.

Abdomen: Soft and nontender to palpation. Bowel sounds are present and no masses or organomegaly are noted.

Extremities: There is no cyanosis, clubbing, or edema. Pulses are +2 and symmetrical in all areas.

Lab Data

Chest Radiograph: See Figure 8-3.

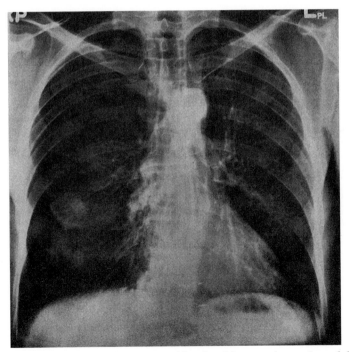

Figure 8-3. Chest radiograph of a 35-year-old male with acute chest pain and dyspnea.

Questions for Case #3

1. Describe the breath sounds heard on auscultation.
2. What pulmonary disorders can cause this patient's problem?
3. What information supports the most likely diagnosis for this patient's problems over the other possibilities?
4. What is the most likely diagnosis?
5. What physiologic principles underlie the auscultatory findings in this case?
6. What abnormalities are seen on the chest radiograph?

Case #4

History of Present Illness

A 40-year-old man has received care on the surgical unit for approximately 5 days after a cholecystectomy. Forty-eight hours previously, he had experienced a sudden onset of dyspnea while in the bathroom. The dyspnea gradually decreased in severity; however, he developed chest pain on the right side approximately 24 hours later. He denies cough, fever, night sweats, or sputum production. He denies leg tenderness or swelling as well as any history of asthma, hay fever, allergies, or wheezing.

Past Medical History

Illnesses: Mild systemic hypertension.

Familial Illnesses: Father and two older brothers died of cardiac arrest.

Occupational History: The patient has worked as an auto mechanic, where he was exposed to brake dust and degreasing solution fumes on a regular basis.

Pets: Goats and sheep kept in the back yard.

Travel: A recent trip to Yellowstone National Park by automobile.

Hobbies: Tending to goats and sheep.

Surgeries: Appendectomy and recent cholecystectomy.

Marital Status: Married to his third wife for 6 years.

Medications: Hydrochlorothiazide.

Smoking History: 20 pack years.

Allergies: None noted.

Physical Examination

General: The patient is an obese male who appears approximately his stated age of 40. He is alert and oriented but mildly dyspneic while lying in bed during the examination.

Vital Signs: Temperature: 38° C; heart rate: 98/min; respiratory rate: 28/min; blood pressure: 120/70 mm Hg.

HEENT: Examination is noncontributory for the current pulmonary problem.

Neck: Trachea is midline and mobile to palpation, and no stridor or wheezing are noted during tidal volume breathing. Carotid pulsations were normal and symmetrical bilaterally; there are no carotid bruits. There is no jugular venous distention or lymphadenopathy noted.

Chest: Normal AP diameter and slightly decreased expansion with respiration.

Heart: Regular rate and rhythm at approximately 98/min apically. No murmurs, heaves, or gallops noted.

Lungs: Refer to Case #4 on the accompanying audio program for the patient's lung sounds.

Abdomen: Soft and nontender to palpation. The recent surgical scar appears to be healing well and is without evidence of inflammation. Bowel sounds are present, and no masses are noted. Urogenital examination is normal.

Extremities: There is no clubbing or edema. Pulses are +2 and symmetrical in all areas. There is no calf tenderness or other evidence of vein inflammation (thrombophlebitis).

Lab Data

ABGs: pH 7.48; $PaCO_2$ 30 mm Hg; PaO_2 55 mm Hg on room air; CBC — WBC = 15,000 mm³; Hgb 14 gm%; Hct 47%; Segs 68%; Bands 4%; Lymphs 28%.

ECG: Shows slight right axis deviation.

Chest Radiograph: See Figure 8-4.

V/Q Lung Scan: Demonstrates a perfusion defect in the right lower lobe with normal ventilation.

Questions for Case #4

1. Describe the breath sounds heard on auscultation.
2. What pulmonary disorders can cause this patient's problem?
3. What information supports the most likely diagnosis for this patient's problems over the other possibilities?
4. What is the most likely diagnosis?
5. What physiologic principles underlie the auscultatory findings in this case?
6. What is your interpretation of the ABG results?
7. What is your interpretation of the chest radiograph?
8. Why does the ECG show right axis deviation?

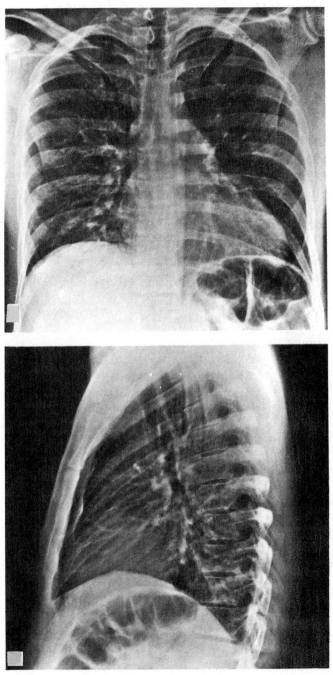

Figure 8-4. Standard PA and lateral chest radiograph, demonstrating increased density in the right lower lobe. The abnormality is more easily seen in the lateral projection.

Case #5

History of Present Illness

The patient is a 25-year-old white female school teacher who presented to the emergency room after a hard day of barrel racing at a local gymkhana event. She complains of severe dyspnea, which began during the vigorous activity associated with her competition. She has been treated for asthma since approximately age 8 with an increasingly complex medication regimen, currently consisting of a beta-agonist metered-dose inhaler (albuterol) used several times daily before exercise and fluticasone (a corticosteroid). She has not recently required oral prednisone. Her current complaints include extreme dyspnea, severe nonproductive cough, a heavy sensation in her chest, and a feeling of impending doom. She has taken all of her medications regularly through the day with the last dose just before her decision to visit the emergency room. She denies recent fever, night sweats, chills, change in sputum, or peripheral edema.

Past Medical History

Illnesses: The patient has been without medical problems except severe asthma. Broken leg at age 12 and broken arm at age 18, both from injuries sustained during horseback competition. Nasal polyps removed at age 20.

Familial Illnesses: None.

Occupational History: High school teacher.

Pets: Four Morgan horses.

Travel: None outside California during the past 2 years.

Hobbies: Horseback competition, grooming shows.

Surgeries: None.

Marital Status: Single.

Medications: Albuterol and fluticasone.

Smoking History: None.

Allergies: Dust, many pollens, aspirin, sulfa drugs, and penicillin.

Physical Examination

General: The patient is a well-developed white female who appears slightly younger than her stated age of 25. She is alert and oriented but is sitting on the edge of the bed with her hands propped on her knees and is complaining of respiratory distress. She is using accessory muscles of respiration and is mildly diaphoretic (sweaty).

Vital Signs: Temperature: 37° C; pulse: 140/min; respirations: 18/min; blood pressure: 160/92 mm Hg. There is a paradoxical pulse of 18 mm Hg.

HEENT: Examination shows slight flaring of the nares with inspiration and cyanosis of the lips.

Neck: Full active range of motion. Trachea is midline and mobile to palpation, and there is no stridor during tidal volume or forced vital capacity maneuvers. There is mild jugular venous distention with respiration. There is no cervical or supraclavicular lymphadenopathy. Carotid pulsations are normal and symmetrical; there are no carotid bruits.

Chest: There is increased AP diameter and decreased expansion with respiration. The chest is resonant to percussion in all lung fields.

Heart: Regular rhythm at 140/min. No murmurs, gallops, rubs, or ventricular heaves.

Lungs: Refer to Case #5 on the audio program for the patient's lung sounds.

Abdomen: Nontender to palpation. The patient is not comfortable lying down, so the abdominal exam was difficult to perform.

Extremities: No clubbing or edema. Cyanosis of the nail beds on both upper and lower extremities. Pulses +2 and symmetrical in all areas.

Lab Data

Pulmonary Function Test: FEV_1 = 1.0 L, FVC = 3.5 L, Peak flow = 105 L/min; ABGs on room air: pH 7.35; $PaCO_2$ 40 mm Hg; PaO_2 40 mm Hg; CBC – WBC = 13,000/mm³; Hgb 13 gm%; Hct 40%; Segs 75%; Bands 5%; Lymphs 20%.

Chest Radiograph: See Figure 8-5, *A* and *B*. The figure shows a chest radiograph typical for this case.

Questions for Case #5

1. Describe the breath sounds heard on auscultation.
2. What pulmonary disorders can cause this patient's problems?
3. What information supports the most likely diagnosis for this patient's problems over the other possibilities?
4. What is the most likely diagnosis?
5. What physiologic principles underlie the auscultatory findings in this case? What could reduce the intensity of the sounds?
6. How do you interpret the ABG results?
7. What is causing the paradoxical pulse, and what is its significance?
8. How do you interpret the chest radiograph?

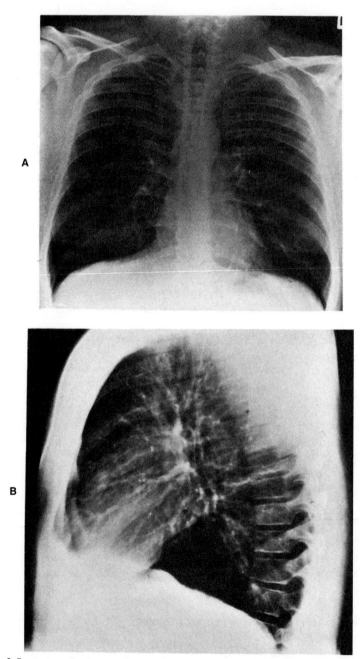

Figure 8-5. A, Standard PA radiograph. **B,** Lateral projection for the same patient.

Case #6

History of Present Illness

The patient is a 64-year-old alcoholic female who has been admitted through the emergency room because of a 2-day history of cough, shaking chills, and sputum production. The sputum is yellow in color, thick, and tenacious. The patient's temperature has been 39° C several times during the 2 days before admission. In addition to the fever, the patient complains of mild dyspnea and severe right lower chest pain during inspiration. The patient has not been eating very well and thinks she has lost about 4 pounds during the week prior to admission. She denies ankle edema, wheezing, palpitations, orthopnea, or paroxysmal nocturnal dyspnea.

Past Medical History

Illnesses: High blood pressure, mild chronic obstructive lung disease.

Familial Illnesses: None.

Occupational History: Retired meatpacker.

Pets: None.

Travel: None.

Hobbies: None.

Surgeries: Removal of basal cell carcinoma of her nose and sigmoid colon polypectomy.

Marital Status: Married 40 years.

Medications: Aspirin, Robitussin, Prozac, and Sudafed.

Smoking History: 40 pack years.

Allergies: None.

Physical Examination

General: The patient is a thin, white female in mild respiratory distress at rest in the hospital bed. She complains primarily of pain in her right chest with respiration. Her mentation is nearly normal; her affect is anxious.

Vital Signs: Temperature: 38.5° C; pulse: 110/min; respirations: 28/min; blood pressure: 150/94 mm Hg.

HEENT: Exam is found to be noncontributory to the present problem.

Neck: Supple with full active range of motion. Trachea midline and mobile to palpation. No stridor is noted during either tidal volume or forced vital capacity maneuvers. Carotid pulsations are +2 and symmetrical, and there are no carotid bruits. There is no cervical or supraclavicular lymphadenopathy and no jugular venous distention.

Chest: Normal anteroposterior diameter, but slightly decreased expansion with respiration, particularly on the right side. There is normal resonance to percussion over most of the chest except the right lower chest, which has decreased resonance.

Heart: Regular rate and rhythm. No murmurs, gallops, or rubs. No ventricular heaves.

Lungs: Refer to Case #6 on the audio program for the patient's lung sounds.

Abdomen: Soft and nontender to palpation. Bowel sounds are present, and the liver is of normal span in the midclavicular line. No masses are noted.

Extremities: There is no cyanosis, clubbing, or edema. Pulses are normal and symmetrical in all areas.

Lab Data

Complete Blood Count: WBC = 24,000/mm³, Hgb 11 gm%, Hct 40%, Segs 80%, Bands 15%, Lymphs 5%.

Chest Radiograph: See Figure 8-6.

Questions for Case #6

1. Describe the breath sounds heard on auscultation.
2. What pulmonary disorders can cause this patient's problem?
3. What information supports the most likely diagnosis for this patient's problem over the other possibilities?
4. What is the most likely diagnosis?
5. What physiologic principles underlie the auscultatory findings in this case?
6. What abnormalities do you see on the chest radiograph? Can you identify the location of any abnormality?
7. How do you interpret the CBC? What is the significance of an elevation in the bands?

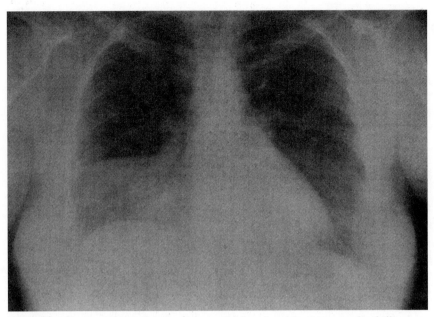

Figure 8-6. Chest radiograph of a 64-year-old female with acute cough, chills, chest pain, and mild dyspnea.

Case #7

History of Present Illness

A 57-year-old male comes to the outpatient clinic complaining of dyspnea with exercise for the past 2 months. He first noticed trouble breathing while walking up inclines on the golf course several months ago and now has difficulty breathing when walking more than 50 feet or so on level ground. He denies cough, sputum production, wheeze, chest pain, or hemoptysis.

Past Medical History

Illnesses: Denies any previous health problems.

Familial Illnesses: Father died of a heart attack at age 60; mother died at age 68 of pulmonary embolism; no brothers or sisters.

Occupational History: Stockbroker for the past 20 years.

Pets: Two ferrets.

Travel: Hawaii each winter.

Hobbies: Golf.

Surgeries: Hernia repair 10 years ago.

Marital Status: Single.

Medications: None.

Smoking History: 30 pack years; quit smoking about 10 years ago.

ETOH History: Drinks a six pack of beer almost every day since the age of 20 years.

Allergies: None.

Physical Examination

General: Well-developed, well-nourished male in no acute distress at rest in the exam room. He is oriented to time, place, and person, has a good memory, and is a good historian.

Vital Signs: Normal at rest.

HEENT: Noncontributory.

Neck: Short, thick neck; trachea is midline and mobile. No stridor or wheezing is noted. Carotid pulses normal bilaterally. Jugular venous distension is not visible. No lymphadenopathy.

Chest: Normal A-P diameter. Normal contour. Good bilateral expansion with deep breathing.

Heart: PMI is not appreciated. Refer to Case #7 on the audio program for this patient's heart sounds.

Lungs: Breath sounds reveal fine late-inspiratory crackles in the bases.

Abdomen: Soft, nontender; bowel sounds present; moderate obesity.

Extremities: Trace edema, warm and dry; no cyanosis or digital clubbing noted; pulses $++$ bilaterally.

Lab Data

Chest Radiograph: Mildly enlarged heart with bilateral interstitial infiltrates.

Complete Blood Count: Normal.

Chemistry Profile: Normal.

Questions for Case #7

1. Describe the heart sounds heard on the audio program for Case #7.
2. What relationship does the abnormal heart sound have with the findings on the chest radiograph and the patient's dyspnea?
3. What physiologic abnormality caused the abnormal heart sound?
4. What disorders are possible causes of the abnormal heart sound?
5. What lifestyle issue in this patient could cause the patient's problem and result in the abnormal heart sounds?
6. Why is jugular venous distension not appreciated in this patient?

📚 Case #8

History of Present Illness

The patient is a 40-year-old female who had an episode of syncope while getting out of the bath tub last night. She awakened on the floor of the bathroom unaware of the expired time but was not injured. She admits to mild dyspnea with exercise and dull chest pain but denies cough, sputum production, hemoptysis, chest pain, leg and ankle swelling, or wheezing.

Past Medical History

Illnesses: None.

Familial Illnesses: Parents are both alive and well; one brother with a history of lung cancer and one sister who is currently well.

Occupational History: Housewife for the past 15 years.

Pets: One dog and two cats at home.

Travel: Has not been out of the country for the past 7 years. Previously visited sister in Canada once per year.

Hobbies: Painting.

Surgeries: Tonsilectomy at age 6.

Marital Status: Married.

Medications: None.

Smoking History: Negative.

Allergies: None.

Physical Examination

General: Alert and oriented to time, place, and person; appears her stated age and in no acute distress at rest.

Vital signs: Normal.

HEENT: Noncontributory.

Neck: No bruits, no JVD, no lymphadenopathy; carotid pulses are equal bilaterally and normal for intensity.

Chest: Normal chest configuration.

Heart: Refer to Case #8 on the audio program for the heart sounds for this patient. The heart sounds are heard over the second intercostal space just to the left of the sternal border. A heave is noted near the right sternal border at the fifth intercostal space.

Lungs: Lung sounds are normal bilaterally.

Abdomen: Normal.

Extremities: Normal.

Lab Data

Complete Blood Count: Normal.

Chest Radiograph: P-A view appears normal; lateral view shows an enlarged right ventricle with a small retrosternal airspace.

Questions for Case #8
1. What abnormal heart sound do you hear?
2. What pathophysiology may explain the abnormal heart sound?
3. How is the abnormal heart sound related to the patient's dyspnea and syncope?
4. What is the differential diagnosis of problems that could cause this abnormal heart sound?
5. What treatment is available for this patient?
6. Why is it important to recognize the abnormal heart sound in this case?
7. Why is the abnormal heart sound best appreciated at the second intercostal space near the sternal border on the left?
8. What is causing the heave at the right sternal border?

📖 Case #9

History of Present Illness

A 68-year-old female presents to the outpatient clinic complaining of shortness of breath and dizziness with stair climbing. The onset of dyspnea is very predictable at the level of the sixth step. Her symptoms have gradually increased over the past several months and are now to the point that she is "afraid something is wrong." She denies wheezing, cough, sputum, hemoptysis, chest pain, and pedal edema.

Past Medical History

Family Illnesses: Mother died of breast cancer, one sister alive and well.

Occupational History: Worked as an accountant for 30 years, currently retired.

Pets: One cat.

Travel: Visits relatives in Florida once a year.

Hobbies: Golf and walking.

Surgeries: Hysterectomy 16 years ago.

Marital Status: Married.

Medications: None.

Smoking History: Negative.

Allergies: None.

Physical Examination

General: Elderly female in no apparent distress at rest. Good memory and good historian.

Vital Signs: Slight tachycardia but otherwise normal.

HEENT: Normal.

Neck: Bruit heard over both carotid arteries.

Chest: Lung sounds clear to auscultation. Normal chest configuration and bilateral expansion noted with deep breathing.

Heart: Refer to Case #9 on the audio program. The heart sound is loudest at the sternal border on the right at the second intercostal space.

Lungs: Lung sounds normal.

Abdomen: Normal.

Extremities: No clubbing or edema; peripheral pulses are weak to palpation.

Lab Data

CBC: Normal.

Chemistry Profile: Normal.

Chest Radiograph: Lungs are clear and heart size is within normal limits.

Questions for Case #9

1. What abnormal heart sound is present in this patient?
2. What causes the abnormal heart sound in this case?
3. How do we know the abnormal heart sound in this case is not due to mitral regurgitation?
4. Why is the abnormality heard also in the carotid arteries?
5. Why is the dyspnea and dizziness so predictable at six stairs?
6. Why does the chest radiograph not show cardiac enlargement in this case?
7. What is the differential diagnosis for causes of this problem?

📚 Case #10

History of Present Illness

The patient is a 44-year-old female who has been noticing shortness of breath while doing housework for several months. She has smoked an average of one pack of cigarettes per day for the past 20 years or so. She only coughs up phlegm when she has a respiratory infection. She denies chest pain, wheezing, fever, and hemoptysis.

Past Medical History

Illnesses: Scarlet fever at the age of 8 years.

Familial Illnessess: Both parents are alive and well; there are no siblings.

Occupational History: Housewife.

Pets: One canary.

Travel: Occasional trips to a local lake for sailing.

Hobbies: Photography.

Surgeries: None.

Marital Status: Married.

Medications: None.

Smoking History: 20 pack years.

Allergies: Penicillin.

Physical Examination

General: Alert, cooperative, well-developed, thin, and in no acute distress at rest.

Vital signs: BP: 118/76 mm Hg; HR: 96/min; RR: 16/min; body temperature: 98.5° F.

HEENT: Noncontributory.

Neck: No thyromegaly; not using accessory muscles with spontaneous breathing; no jugular venous distention; no carotid bruits.

Chest: Normal in appearance.

Heart: Refer to Case #10 on the audio program for the heart sounds in this case.

Lungs: Normal breath sound bilaterally.

Abdomen: Normal.

Extremities: No edema.

Lab Data

Chest Radiograph: Heart size is at the upper limits of normal; lung fields are clear.

ECG: Changes consistent with left atrial enlargement.

Questions for Case #10

1. Describe the abnormal heart sound heard on the audio program for Case #10.
2. Does the abnormal heart sound help explain the ECG abnormality?
3. How does the abnormal heart sound help explain the dyspnea?
4. What is the most likely cause of the heart abnormality responsible for the abnormal heart sound?
5. Is this abnormal heart sound best heard with the bell or the diaphragm of the stethoscope?

ANSWERS TO QUESTIONS FOR CASE STUDIES

Answers and Discussion for Case #1

Purpose of Case: To differentiate between asthma and emphysema, based on loudness of breath sounds and other findings.

Diagnosis: Emphysema caused by alpha-1 antitrypsin deficiency.

1. **Describe the breath sounds heard from Case #1 on the accompanying audio program.**
   Breath sounds are very quiet in all lung fields, and there is no evidence of stridor, wheezing, or crackles.
2. **What pulmonary disorders can cause this patient's problem?**
   Severe asthma, cystic fibrosis, and emphysema.
3. **What information supports the most likely diagnosis for this patient's problems over the other possibilities?**
   The patient's diminished breath sounds (with no crackles or wheezes during normal breathing) are evidence against asthma and cystic fibrosis. Her physical exam and chest radiograph reveal pulmonary hyperexpansion. The patient's familial history of obstructive lung disease (occurring in her father at a young age) increases the likelihood of hereditary emphysema.
4. **What is the most likely diagnosis?**
   Emphysema caused by alpha-1 antitrypsin deficiency (also called genetic emphysema).
5. **What physiologic principles underlie the auscultatory findings in this case?**
   This patient with alpha-1 antitrypsin deficiency has lost elastic recoil in her lungs; therefore distal bronchioles collapse during early expiration, trapping air in the lungs. As a result, the lungs become hyperexpanded. The airways obstruction severely limits airflow throughout the bronchial tree, thus preventing the development of turbulence and reducing sound production. In addition, hyperexpanded lung fields transmit sounds poorly. The result is diminished lung and heart sounds.
6. **Are the breath sounds consistent with the pulmonary function test results?**
   Yes, the PFT results demonstrate obstructive lung disease that results in pulmonary hyperinflation and reduced transmission of breath sounds to the chest wall.
7. **What abnormalities are present on the chest radiograph?**
   The chest radiograph shows severe pulmonary hyperinflation. The lateral view shows an increased retrosternal airspace typical of emphysema. The vascular markings are absent in the lower lung fields, which is consistent with alpha-1 antitrypsin deficiency.

Answers and Discussion for Case #2

Purpose of Case: To differentiate lower from upper airway obstruction based on type of wheeze and radiation of the sounds.

Diagnosis: Laryngeal carcinoma.

1. **Describe the breath sounds heard on auscultation over the neck.**
   At the neck there is stridor present during inspiration.
2. **What pulmonary disorders can cause this patient's problem?**
   Epiglottitis, foreign body aspiration, asthma, and partial upper airway obstruction from tumor or anatomic defect.
3. **What information supports the most likely diagnosis for this patient's problems over the other possibilities?**
   The lack of response to bronchodilators, the brassy progressive cough, the monophonic nature of the wheeze, and the uniform distribution of the wheeze heard best over the upper airway and gradually diminishing in intensity toward the bases make this more likely a single-source wheeze. (Multiple notes would be expected to occur in asthma, with many small airways vibrating.) Symptoms of epiglottitis would be of acute onset.
4. **What is the most likely diagnosis?**
   Partial upper airway obstruction.
5. **What physiologic principles underlie the auscultatory findings in this case?**
   Wheezing and stridor are produced by vibration of the airway wall. The pitch of the sound is determined by the characteristics of the vibrating wall of the airway and is independent of the diameter or length of the airway in which the vibrations occur. Because mass and elasticity of the bronchial wall determine the note produced when it vibrates, a disease affecting many bronchi of varying sizes would produce a polyphonic wheeze as opposed to a disease affecting only one bronchus, the larynx, or the trachea. The wheeze or stridor of upper airway obstruction is more prominent during inspiration in many cases because it is extrathoracic in origin and is loudest over the neck (see Chapter 6).
6. **What pathophysiology may explain the flow-volume loop results?**
   Nonfixed narrowing of the extrathoracic airway worsens with inspiratory efforts because the upper airway is not surrounded or affected by pleural pressures. The marked reduction in inspiratory flows is consistent with extrathoracic airway narrowing. There is minimal reduction of expiratory flows.
7. **What procedure should be done next to diagnose the patient's problem?**
   Bronchoscopy.

Answers and Discussion for Case #3

Purpose of Case: To demonstrate abnormalities associated with pneumothorax.

Diagnosis: Pneumothorax on right side.

1. **Describe the breath sounds heard on auscultation.**
   There are diminished breath sounds on the right side and normal breath sounds on the left side of the chest. There are no wheezes or crackles.

2. **What pulmonary disorders can cause this patient's problem?**
   Spontaneous pneumothorax, aspirated foreign body, pneumonia, or pulmonary embolus.

3. **What information supports the most likely diagnosis for this patient's problems over the other possibilities?**
   The sudden onset of chest pain and dyspnea points to an acute event. The asymmetrical chest with diminished respiratory excursions on the right side would be consistent with the pneumothorax. Increased resonance to percussion on the right side is compatible with excess air in the right thoracic cavity. Decreased breath sounds on the larger side indicate either absence of airflow in that bronchial tree or acoustical attenuation between the bronchial tree and the chest wall—or both.

4. **What is the most likely diagnosis?**
   Spontaneous right pneumothorax.

5. **What physiologic principles underlie the auscultatory findings in this case?**
   The elastic recoil of the lung normally counterbalances the tendency of the ribs to expand. When a pneumothorax occurs, the pulmonary elastic recoil is lost, and the chest wall expands unopposed. If a substantial amount of air leaks out of the lung and accumulates in the thoracic space, the mediastinal structures can be pushed toward the other side (tension pneumothorax), thus causing the trachea to deviate toward the opposite side away from the pneumothorax. The absence of lung expansion with respiration on the side of the pneumothorax would decrease ventilation and sound generation on that side; the large accumulation of air within the pleural space would attenuate breath sounds generated in the larger airways.

6. **What abnormalities are seen on the chest radiograph?**
   The chest radiograph shows partial collapse of the right lung. The pleural lining of the right lung is visible. The mediastinal contents are shifted to the left as a result of the pneumothorax on the right.

Answers and Discussion for Case #4

Purpose of Case: To demonstrate pleural friction rub.

Diagnosis: Pulmonary embolus.

1. **Describe the breath sounds heard on auscultation.**
   Normal breath sounds with an inspiratory and expiratory pleural friction rub.

2. **What pulmonary disorders can cause this patient's problem?**
   Pneumonia or pulmonary embolus.

3. **What information supports the most likely diagnosis for this patient's problems over the other possibilities?**
   The diagnosis is indicated by the predisposing factors, surgery, and bed rest, associated with the sudden onset of dyspnea during exercise. The evidence for pulmonary embolus is strengthened by the pleural friction rub, although that could also occur with pneumonia. The ABG results that show hypocapnia and hypoxemia, fever, and leukocytosis can all be seen with both pulmonary embolus and pneumonia. The chest radiograph does not show any signs of pneumonia or pneumothorax. A $\dot{V}/\dot{Q}$ lung scan was needed to confirm the diagnosis of pulmonary embolism. With pneumonia, both ventilation and perfusion are generally impaired in the affected region. When there is impaired perfusion in the affected region and ventilation is normal, there is a high probability of pulmonary embolism. Sometimes, however, both ventilation and perfusion are abnormal, and a pulmonary angiogram or angiographic chest CT is necessary to prove that a pulmonary embolus is present.

4. **What is the most likely diagnosis?**
   Pulmonary embolus.

5. **What physiologic principles underlie the auscultatory findings in this case?**
   The affected pleural surface becomes inflamed. The visceral pleura no longer slides freely over the parietal pleura but rather moves in small increments, thus producing many discrete discontinuous sounds or crackles, much like the sound produced by rubbing two inflated balloons together.

6. **What is your interpretation of the ABG results?**
   The ABG results demonstrate an acute respiratory alkalosis with moderate hypoxemia on room air. Both pneumonia and pulmonary embolism could cause such results.

7. **What is your interpration of the chest radiograph?**
   The chest radiograph appears normal. Common abnormalities seen with pulmonary embolism include subsegmented atelectasis, elevated diaphragm, and small pleural effusion. Westermark's sign may be seen

in some chest radiographs when pulmonary embolism is present. This sign is seen as a paucity of blood vessels in the affected area, caused by obstruction of blood flow by the clot. Although these signs are absent in this patient's chest radiograph, pulmonary embolism remains the most likely diagnosis.

8. Why does the ECG show right axis deviation?

Pulmonary embolism puts a strain on the right ventricle as it attempts to pump blood through the partially occluded pulmonary vasculature. This strain causes the ECG axis to shift from left to right.

Answers and Discussion for Case #5

Purpose of Case: To demonstrate wheezing during severe bronchospasm.

Diagnosis: Severe asthma.

1. **Describe the breath sounds heard on auscultation.**

   There are inspiratory crackles with severe expiratory polyphonic wheezing.

2. **What pulmonary disorders can cause this patient's problems?**

   Exacerbation of the patient's asthma, pulmonary embolus, pneumonia, or bronchitis.

3. **What information supports the most likely diagnosis for this patient's problems over the other possibilities?**

   Diagnosis is indicated by the history of asthma requiring multiple daily medications. Also, the patient's asthma worsens rather suddenly during an activity associated with exposure to dust and animal dander.

4. **What is the most likely diagnosis?**

   Status asthmaticus.

5. **What physiologic principles underlie the auscultatory findings in this case? What could reduce the intensity of the sounds?**

   Production of wheezing depends on bronchial wall vibration, which is produced by rapid airflow through a partially obstructed airway. In this case, the patient is still able to generate sufficient airflow to produce loud wheezing. When airflow within the bronchus is sufficiently diminished, it no longer affects the bronchial wall enough to cause vibration, and wheezing diminishes. With extreme airway obstruction, airflow may be so impaired that wheezing disappears. Bronchodilation could also result in reduced intensity of the wheezing. Careful assessment of numerous parameters is needed to interpret the changes in lung sounds.

6. **How do you interpret the ABG results?**

   The ABG results show severe hypoxemia on room air. The $PaCO_2$ of 40 mm Hg is usually an indication of normal ventilation; however, in this case the $PaCO_2$ is expected to be low during an acute asthma attack. The $PaCO_2$ of 40 mm Hg represents an early warning sign of fatigue and respiratory failure.

7. **What is causing the paradoxical pulse, and what is its significance?**

   Paradoxical pulse occurs when the muscles of breathing are working hard to cause ventilation. Strong inspiratory efforts cause the pleural pressure to drop significantly. The extreme negative intrathoracic pressure that occurs with each inspiratory effort causes an intermittent impedance to blood flow out of the thorax. As a result, the peripheral pulse pressure drops with each coinciding systole. The significance of paradoxical pulse lies in its suggestion of a more severe case of asthma.

8. **How do you interpret the chest radiograph?**

The chest radiograph shows hyperinflation of the lungs. The lateral view shows a low, flat diaphragm and a large retrosternal air space.

Answers and Discussion for Case #6

Purpose of Case: To demonstrate lung sound changes associated with lobar consolidation.

Diagnosis: Lobar pneumonia in right lower lobe.

1. **Describe the breath sounds heard on auscultation.**
   There are bronchial breath sounds limited to the right anterior lower chest.

2. **What pulmonary disorders can cause this patient's problem?**
   Pneumonia, bronchogenic carcinoma, and pulmonary embolus.

3. **What information supports the most likely diagnosis for this patient's problem over the other possibilities?**
   The clinical history of fever, chills, sputum production, dyspnea, and chest pain in an alcoholic are most consistent with pneumonia. The breath sounds reveal the typical findings associated with lung consolidation, including bronchial breathing and egophony.

4. **What is the most likely diagnosis?**
   Pneumonia (sputum culture grew *Streptococcus pneumoniae*).

5. **What physiologic principles underlie the auscultatory findings in this case?**
   Sound is transmitted readily through the airways. The frequencies above 200 HTZ are filtered by normal lung tissue at a rate of 15 decibels per octave. Breath sounds depend on turbulence in the large airways and are predominantly a high-frequency sound. Spoken sounds are also high frequency. Lung consolidation provides a direct path for sound transmission from the larger airways to the chest wall. This allows turbulent airflow sounds in the bronchus, whispered sounds, and spoken sounds to be transmitted to the chest wall with more intensity and clarity.

6. **What abnormalities do you see on the chest radiograph? Can you identify the location of any abnormality?**
   The chest radiograph demonstrates a consolidation in the right middle lobe typical of pneumonia. The location of the pneumonia is verified by the fact that the right heart border is not visible. Because the right middle lobe is anterior in the chest in the same plane as the heart, consolidation in the right middle lobe will cause the right heart border to be invisible.

7. **How do you interpret the CBC? What is the significance of an elevation in the bands?**
   The CBC shows mild anemia, a markedly elevated white cell count and marked elevation of segmented and banded neutrophils. The elevated band count suggests significant stress on the bone marrow, which is releasing immature white cells to combat the pneumonia.

Answers and Discussion for Case #7

Purpose of Case: To demonstrate the heart sounds associated with cardiomegaly.

Diagnosis: Cardiomegaly due to abuse of alcohol.

1. Describe the heart sounds heard on the audio program for Case #7.
   The heart sounds for this case reveal an S3 gallop.
2. What relationship does the abnormal heart sound have with the findings on the chest radiograph and the patient's dyspnea?
   The S3 gallop is consistent with cardiomegaly from an enlarged left ventricle and the infiltrates are probably the result of fluid backing up into the lung (i.e., congestive heart failure), which often leads to dyspnea.
3. What physiologic abnormality caused the abnormal heart sound?
   A stiff left ventricle and the sudden deceleration of blood entering the ventricle.
4. What disorders are possible causes of the abnormal heart sound?
   Ischemic cardiomegaly, viral cardiomegaly, cardiomegaly due to alcohol abuse, and idiopathic cardiomegaly are all possible causes.
5. What lifestyle issue in this patient could cause the patient's problem and result in the abnormal heart sounds?
   Abuse of alcohol leads to cardiomegaly in some patients. This causes congestive heart failure and a stiff left ventricle, which in turn leads to the S3 gallop.
6. Why is jugular venous distention not appreciated in this patient?
   Venous distension is difficult to see in patients with a short, thick neck.

Answers and Discussion for Case #8

Purpose of Case: To demonstrate the importance of identifying a loud P-2.

Diagnosis: Primary pulmonary hypertension.

1. What abnormal heart sound do you hear?
   A loud P-2 is heard.
2. What pathophysiology may explain the abnormal heart sound?
   Forceful closure of the pulmonic valve from pulmonary hypertension is the most likely explanation.
3. How is the abnormal heart sound related to the patient's dyspnea and syncope?
   Pulmonary hypertension is known to cause shortness of breath and may cause syncope in advanced stages.
4. What is the differential diagnosis of problems that could cause this abnormal heart sound?
   Primary pulmonary hypertension, diet pill use, chronic pulmonary embolism, and collagen vascular disease.
5. What treatment is available for this patient?
   Three treatments are available: 1) IV or oral pulmonary vasodilator therapy; 2) oxygen therapy; and 3) lung transplant.
6. Why is it important to recognize the abnormal heart sound in this case?
   Because the patient could die from primary pulmonary hypertension without treatment if the diagnosis is not recognized.
7. Why is the abnormal heart sound best appreciated at the second intercostal space near the sternal border on the left?
   It is best appreciated here because this is where the pulmonic valve is best evaluated (see Chapter 4).
8. What is causing the heave at the right sternal border?
   Right ventricular hypertrophy.

Answers and Discussion for Case #9

Purpose of Case: To differentiate between systolic ejection murmurs and regurgitation murmurs.

Diagnosis: Aortic stenosis that presents with a systolic ejection murmur.

1. **What abnormal heart sound is present in this patient?**
   A systolic ejection murmur is heard.

2. **What causes the abnormal heart sound in this case?**
   Turbulent blood flow through a stenotic aortic or pulmonic valve could cause the murmur heard in this case. Because the murmur is also heard over the carotid arteries in the neck and is loudest at the second right intercostal space at the sternal border, it is most likely due to aortic stenosis.

3. **How do we know the abnormal heart sound in this case is not due to mitral regurgitation?**
   The weak pulses peripherally and the radiation of the murmur to the neck both suggest aortic stenosis. Also, the murmur of mitral valve regurgitation is pansystolic in most cases.

4. **Why is the abnormality heard also in the carotid arteries?**
   The carotid arteries are directly downstream from the aorta and the sound is transmitted along the aorta to the carotid artery.

5. **Why is the dyspnea and dizziness so predictable at six stairs?**
   The stenosis limits blood flow from the heart to the muscles. The muscles become ischemic at a predictable and consistent workload.

6. **Why does the chest radiograph not show cardiac enlargement in this case?**
   The problem is probably in its early stages. The heart will enlarge if the patient is not treated (probably with aortic valve replacement).

7. **What is the differential diagnosis for causes of this problem?**
   Congenital aortic stenosis, rheumatic heart disease, and senile aortic stenosis are possible causes.

Answers and Discussion for Case #10

Purpose of Case: To demonstrate the abnormal heart sound of mitral stenosis.

Diagnosis: Mitral stenosis caused by rheumatic fever as a child.

1. **Describe the abnormal heart sound heard on the audio program for Case #10.**
   This is a diastolic murmur (i.e., starts after the second heart sound and ends before the first heart sound). The sound is caused by blood flowing from the atrium into the ventricle through a narrowed atrial-ventricular valve.

2. **Does the abnormal heart sound help explain the ECG abnormality?**
   Yes. Left atrial enlargement develops as a result of increased pressure in the left atrium from the resistance created by a narrowed mitral valve.

3. **How does the abnormal heart sound help explain the dyspnea?**
   Mitral stenosis impairs the flow of blood from the left atrium into the left ventricle, thus leading to a reduction in the cardiac output. Shortness of breath occurs as a result of impaired delivery of oxygen to the muscles during exertion.

4. **What is the most likely cause of the heart abnormality responsible for the abnormal heart sound?**
   A history of scarlet fever as a child makes mitral valve stenosis resulting from rheumatic fever (i.e., rheumatic heart disease) very likely.

5. **Is the abnormal heart sound best heard with the bell or the diaphragm of the stethoscope?**
   The murmur of mitral valve stenosis is described as a low-pitched diastolic rumble. Low-pitched sounds are best heard with the bell of the stethoscope pressed lightly against the chest, whereas high-pitched sounds are best heard with the diaphragm (see Chapter 4).

Glossary of Key Terms

absorption – the transfer of energy from the sound wave to the obstructing tissue.

acoustical impedence – the resistance offered by the medium (tissue) to the passage of sound.

adventitious lung sounds – abnormal lung sounds superimposed on the breath sounds. They are described as crackles, wheezes, or stridor.

afterload – the resistance to blood flow out of the left ventricle during systole.

apical impulse – the normal pulsation created on the anterior chest with left ventricular contraction.

attenuation – the decrease in the energy of sound as it travels through time and space.

barrel chest – abnormal anterior-posterior (A-P) enlargement of the chest cage due to a loss of lung recoil and hyperinflation. Most often seen in patients with emphysema.

binaural – stethoscope that employs two earpieces in the process of auscultation.

Bowles – the first model of stethoscope to employ a diaphragm in the chestpiece.

bronchial breath sounds – abnormal breath sounds heard over the peripheral chest that have equal inspiratory and expiratory components and are louder and higher pitched than the normal vesicular breath sounds.

bronchophony – an increase in voice sounds heard over the peripheral chest with a stethoscope due to lung consolidation.

bulging – abnormal protruding of the skin between the ribs during forceful exhalation.

C

Cammann – the first model of stethoscope with a binaural design.

cardiac output – the amount of blood pumped out of the left ventricle each minute. Reported in liters per minute.

clubbing – abnormal enlargement of the distal portion of the digits with curvature of the fingernails.

compressional wave – a transient increase in air pressure moving away from the sound source during the propagation of a sound wave.

contractility – a measure of the ability of the heart muscle to contract forcefully.

copious – refers to a large amount, as in a large amount of sputum production.

cor pulmonale – right heart failure due to chronic lung disease.

costochondritis – inflammation of the cartilage connecting the ribs to the sternum.

cough – a forceful expiratory maneuver designed to expel phlegm and foreign material from the lung.

crackles – a discontinuous adventitious lung sound.

crepitation – a historical term used in the past to describe discontinuous adventitious lung sounds.

cyanosis – a bluish discoloration of the skin or mucous membranes caused by reduced oxygenation of the hemoglobin.

D

diaphragm – the major muscle of inspiration. Separates the abdominal contents from the thoracic contents.

diastole – the normal period during the cardiac cycle in which the ventricles relax.

dyspnea – shortness of breath as perceived by the patient.

E

egophony – a change in the spoken voice as perceived over the peripheral chest during auscultation due to lung consolidation. The voice sound takes on a nasal quality that is higher pitched.

ejection fraction – the percent of end diastolic volume pumped out of the left ventricle during systole.

F

fremitus – vibrations felt over the peripheral chest as the patient is asked to repeat a phrase such as "ninety-nine."

frequency – the number of cycles per second created by a sound wave.

G

gallop rhythm – the heart sound associated with the presence of abnormal added sounds (S3/S4).

H

heave – abnormal pulsation on the anterior chest wall often caused by hypertrophy of the left or right ventricle.
hemoptysis – coughing up blood or bloody sputum from the lung.
hepatomegaly – abnormal enlargement of the liver.
Hertz – a measure of sound wave frequency in cycles per second.

I

intensity – the degree of sound wave amplitude.
intimate space – the immediate space around the patient (up to 18 inches) most useful for the physical examination.

J

jugular venous distension – engorgement of the veins in the neck, most often due to right heart failure.

L

Laennec – the French physician credited with developing the first stethoscope.
lift – abnormal pulsation on the anterior chest due to hypertrophy of the heart.
Littmann – a current manufacturer of modern stethoscopes.
lymphadenopathy – abnormal enlargement of the lymph nodes; often occurs with infection and malignancy.

M

megahertz – one million cycles per second.
monaural stethoscope – single tube–designed stethoscope.
murmurs – abnormal heart sounds created by the movement of blood through defective heart valves.

O

orthopnea – difficult breathing in the reclining position or better breathing in the upright position.

P

paradoxical pulse – a significant drop in pulse pressure with each inspiration.

parietal pleura – the layer of the pleura attached to the chest wall.

paroxysmal nocturnal dyspnea – the sudden onset of shortness of breath during sleep.

pectus carinatum – abnormal protrusion of the sternum.

pectus excavatum – abnormal retraction of the sternum.

pericardial friction rub – an abnormal heart sound produced by the rubbing together of the myocardium and pericardium during contraction and relaxation of the ventricles, most often due to inflammation.

personal space – the area around the patient most useful for the interview (2 to 4 feet).

physiologic murmur – a murmur created by rapid blood flow through a healthy valve.

Piorry – an early design of monaural stethoscopes.

pitch – the subjective perception of sound frequency.

platypnea – shortness of breath in the upright position.

pleural friction rub – the abnormal sound created by the rubbing together of the two layers of the pleura when inflammation is present.

point of maximum impulse (PMI) – the pulsation created by left ventricular contraction on the anterior chest wall.

precordium – the area on the chest wall overlying the heart.

preload – the volume of blood filling the ventricle just prior to contraction.

purulent – containing pus.

R

rales – the original term used by Laennec to describe abnormal lung sounds.

reflection – the reversal of sound wave direction due to the presence of an obstacle.

resonance – the normal sound created when the chest wall is percussed to detect underlying lung condition. The sound is similar to that created when tapping on a drum.

respiration – the process of gas exchange between the lung and blood (external) or between the blood and tissues (internal).

retractions – abnormal sinking inward of the skin between the ribs with each inspiration; its presence signifies a large drop in pleural pressure during inspiration and signifies a large increase in the work of breathing.

rhonchi – a term used to describe low-pitched continuous type of adventitious lung sounds. Because the term has been used in the past for a variety of sounds, its use is not recommended.

S

S1 – the abbreviation for the first heart sound.

S2 – the abbreviation for the second heart sound.

S3 – the abbreviation for a third heart sound. It occurs early in diastole just after S2.

S4 – the abbreviation for a fourth heart sound. It occurs late in diastole just before S1.

social space – the distance from the patient in which an introduction is appropriate (approximately 4 to 12 feet from the patient).

sound wave – the propagation of compressional waves in a sequential manner through the conducting medium.

split S1 – the sound created when the mitral and tricuspid valves do not close simultaneously.

split S2 – the sound created when the pulmonic and aortic valves do not close simultaneously.

stethoscope – a device used to auscultate the heart and lungs.

stridor – an abnormal continuous adventitious lung sound heard over the upper airway; it indicates partial obstruction of the airway.

stroke volume – the volume of blood ejected by the left ventricle during each systole.

subsonic sound – sound waves occurring below 20 Htz.

systole – the normal period of the cardiac cycle associated with ventricular contraction.

T

thrills – abnormal vibrations felt over the heart related to the rapid movement of blood through a narrowed opening.

tracheal breath sounds – the sounds of breathing heard over the trachea.

tracheobronchial tree – the airways designed to conduct gas to and from the lungs.

U

ultrasonic sound – sound waves with a frequency above 20,000 Htz, not detectable by the human ear.

V

ventilation – the movement of air in and out of the lung with breathing.

vesicular breath sounds – the normal sounds of breathing heard over the peripheral lung areas.

visceral pleura – the layer of the pleura attached to the lung.

W

wheeze – a continuous type of adventitious lung sound. Most often indicates narrowing of the intrathoracic airways.

whispered pectoriloquy – alteration in the spoken whispered voice as perceived over the peripheral chest during auscultation due to con-solidation of the lung.

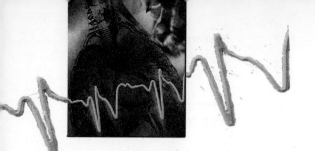

Answer Key for Review Questions

CHAPTER 1

1. c
2. b
3. d
4. true
5. true
6. false
7. a
8. true
9. false
10. b
11. false
12. true

CHAPTER 2

1. d
2. a
3. c
4. true
5. false
6. d
7. a
8. c
9. true
10. true
11. a
12. b
13. c
14. b

CHAPTER 3

1. false
2. true
3. false
4. true
5. false
6. true
7. true
8. false
9. true
10. false
11. c
12. b
13. d
14. d
15. d

CHAPTER 4

1. b
2. c
3. b
4. a
5. b
6. d
7. b
8. a
9. d
10. true
11. false
12. a
13. c
14. b
15. b

CHAPTER 5

1. a
2. d
3. c
4. b
5. a
6. b

7. c
8. true

CHAPTER 6

1. d
2. a
3. d
4. true
5. d
6. c
7. d
8. d
9. c
10. c
11. b
12. d
13. a
14. d
15. d
16. a
17. b
18. d
19. a

CHAPTER 7

1. false
2. true
3. false
4. true
5. true
6. true
7. false
8. true
9. d
10. a
11. b
12. b
13. c
14. a
15. a

Lung and Heart Sounds on Audio Program

ADULT LUNG SOUNDS

1. Introduction
2. Tracheobronchial breath sounds
3. Bronchovesicular breath sounds
4. Vesicular breath sounds
5. Diminished breath sounds
6. Bronchial breath sounds heard over lung consolidation (Courtesy of Dr. Roy Donnerberg.)
7. Medium inspiratory crackles
8. Medium inspiratory and expiratory crackles
9. Coarse inspiratory and expiratory crackles
10. Fine, late-inspiratory crackles typical for pulmonary fibrosis
11. Mild expiratory wheeze
12. Inspiratory crackles with moderate expiratory wheezes
13. Inspiratory crackles with severe expiratory wheezes
14. Pleural friction rub (heard on inspiration and expiration)
15. Inspiratory and expiratory stridor
16. Bone crepitus
17. Subcutaneous emphysema
18. Chest hair rubbing against the diaphragm of the stethoscope
19. Normal voice sounds followed by egophony
20. Normal voice sounds followed by bronchophony
21. Normal whispered sound followed by whispered pectoriloquy

INFANT LUNG SOUNDS

22. Tracheobronchial breath sounds
23. Vesicular breath sounds
24. Vesicular breath sounds with crying
25. Stridor
26. Fine inspiratory crackles

27. Medium inspiratory and expiratory crackles
28. Expiratory grunting
29. Inspiratory and expiratory low-pitched wheezes
30. Water in tubing with patient on CPAP system

HEART SOUNDS

31. Normal S1 and S2 at a heart rate of 70 beats/min
32. Normal S1 and S2 at a heart rate of 110 beats/min
33. Normal S1 and split S2
34. S1, S2, and S3
35. S4, S1, and S2
36. Gallop rhythm with both S3 and S4
37. Loud P2 associated with pulmonary hypertension
38. Systolic murmur associated with mitral regurgitation
39. Systolic ejection murmur associated with aortic stenosis (From Tilkian AG, Conover MB: *Understanding heart sounds and murmurs with an introduction to lung sounds,* ed 4, Philadelphia, 2001, Saunders.)
40. Systolic murmur associated with pulmonic stenosis
41. Patent ductus arteriosus heard over the precordium of an infant
42. Pericardial friction rub

LUNG AND HEART SOUNDS FOR CHAPTER 8 CASE STUDIES

The heart sound for Case #10 is from Tilkian AG, Conover MB: *Understanding heart sounds and murmurs with an introduction to lung sounds,* ed 4, Philadelphia, 2001, Saunders.

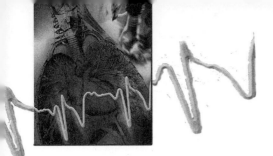

Index

Page numbers followed by *f* indicate figures; *t*, tables.

Hertz (Hz), 31
History
 family, 52
 medical, 43–52
  past, reviewing, 50
 pharmacologic, 52
 of present illness, reviewing, 50
 smoking, 51–52
 social, 52
Hypertension
 pulmonary
  case study on, 138–139, 153
  loud P2 in, 109
  split S2 in, 110
 systemic, loud S2 in, 109
Hypotension, systemic, diminished
  S2 in, 109
Hypovolemia, diminished S2 in,
  108–109

I

Impedance, acoustical,
 of medium, 38
Infants
 lung sounds in, on audio
  program, 165–166
 wheezing in, 94
Inspection
 cardiac, 61
 chest, 52–56
Inspiration, 1
 mechanics of, 9
Intensity, sound, 32, 33f
Intercostal muscle, 8, 8f
Interviewing, fundamentals of,
  43–45
Intimate space, 44, 44f
Inverse square law, sound
  attenuation and, 35, 35f

J

Jugular venous distention, 55, 56f

L

Laennec stethoscope, 69–70, 69f
Laryngeal dysfunction syndrome,
  wheezing in, 95
Laryngeal subglottic stenosis,
  wheezing and, 95
Larynx, 2f, 3
 anatomy of, 2f
 carcinoma of, case study on,
  121–123, 145
 functions of, 3
 obstruction of, stridor in, 95
Left bundle branch block,
  paradoxical splitting of heart
  sounds in, 111
Lift, 62
Littmann stethoscope
 electronic, 74, 75f
 tunable, 74, 74f
Lobar pneumonia, case study on,
  133–134, 135f, 151
Lung(s)
 alterations with chest disease,
  14–15
 anatomy and physiology of, 1–16
 anatomy of, 2–6
 anterior-posterior view of, 12–13,
  12f, 13f
 auscultation of, 56–59, 58f
 function of, 1–2
 lateral view of, 13–14
 parenchyma of, sound
  transmission and, 5–6
 percussion of, 60–61, 61f
 posterior-anterior view of, 13, 13f
Lung sounds, 79–102
 adventitious, 86–96. See
  Adventitious lung sounds.
 on audio program, 165
 infant, on audio program,
  165–166
Lung-thorax, model of, 10f
Lymphadenopathy, 60